Quality

Editors

BARBARA LEEPER
ROSEMARY LUQUIRE

CRITICAL CARE NURSING CLINICS OF NORTH AMERICA

www.ccnursing.theclinics.com

Consulting Editor
JAN FOSTER

December 2014 • Volume 26 • Number 4

ELSEVIER

1600 John F. Kennedy Boulevard • Suite 1800 • Philadelphia, Pennsylvania, 19103-2899

http://www.theclinics.com

CRITICAL CARE NURSING CLINICS OF NORTH AMERICA Volume 26, Number 4
December 2014 ISSN 0899-5885, ISBN-13: 978-0-323-32644-5

Editor: Kerry Holland
Developmental Editor: Stephanie Carter

Critical Care Nursing Clinics of North America (ISSN 0899-5885) is published quarterly by Elsevier Inc., 360 Park Avenue South, New York, NY 10010-1710. Months of issue are March, June, September, and December. Business and Editorial Offices: 1600 John F. Kennedy Blvd., Suite 1800, Philadelphia, PA 19103-2899. Periodicals postage paid at New York, NY and additional mailing offices. Subscription prices are $150.00 per year for US individuals, $328.00 per year for US institutions, $80.00 per year for US students and residents, $200.00 per year for Canadian individuals, $412.00 per year for Canadian institutions, $230.00 per year for international individuals, $412.00 per year for international institutions and $115.00 per year for Canadian and international students/residents. To receive student/resident rate, orders must be accompanied by name of affiliated institution, data of term, and the signature of program/residency coordinator on institution letterhead. Orders will be billed at individual rate until proof of status is received. Foreign air speed delivery is included in all Clinics subscription prices. All prices are subject to change without notice. POSTMASTER: Send address changes to Critical Care Nursing Clinics of North America, Elsevier Health Sciences Division, Subscription Customer Service, 3251 Riverport Lane, Maryland Heights, MO 63043. Customer Service: 1-800-654-2452 (US and Canada); 314-447-8871 (outside US and Canada). Fax: 314-447-8029. E-mail: JournalsCustomerService-usa@elsevier.com (for print support) and JournalsOnlineSupport-usa@elsevier.com (for online support).

Reprints. For copies of 100 or more of articles in this publication, please contact the Commercial Reprints Department, Elsevier Inc., 360 Park Avenue South, New York, New York, 10010-1710; Tel.: 212-633-3874, Fax: 212-633-3820, and E-mail: reprints@elsevier.com.

Critical Care Nursing Clinics of North America is covered in MEDLINE/PubMed (Index Medicus), International Nursing Index, Nursing Citation Index, Cumulative Index to Nursing and Allied Health Literature, and RNdex Top 100.

Contributors

CONSULTING EDITOR

JAN FOSTER, PhD, RN, CNS
Formerly, Associate Professor, College of Nursing, Texas Woman's University, Houston;
Currently, President, Nursing Inquiry and Intervention Inc., The Woodlands, Texas

EDITORS

BARBARA LEEPER, MN, RN-BC, CNS M-S, CCRN, FAHA
Clinical Nurse Specialist, Cardiovascular Services, Baylor University Medical Center at
Dallas, Dallas, Texas

ROSEMARY LUQUIRE, RN, PhD, NEA-BC, FAAN
Senior Vice President and Chief Nursing Executive, Baylor Scott and White Health,
North Texas, Dallas, Texas

AUTHORS

BRIGETTE ADAIR, BSN, RN, CCRN, NE-BC
Nurse Manager, 4 Roberts Intensive Care Unit, Baylor University Medical Center at Dallas,
Dallas, Texas

DENA ALLEN, MSN, RN, PhD(c), CCRN
Nurse Manager of the Cardiothoracic & Heart-Lung Transplant ICU and Coronary Care
Unit, Baylor University Medical Center at Dallas, Dallas, Texas

CHRISTINE BALCH, RN, BSN, OCN
Clinical Supervisor, Department of Nursing, Baylor University Medical Center, T. Boone
Pickens Cancer Hospital, Dallas, Texas

JASMIRY D. BENNETT, MS, RN, ACNP-BC
Baylor Heart and Vascular Hospital, Dallas, Texas

RYAN BESEDA, BSN, RN, CCRN
Department of Critical Care Services, Baylor University Medical Center at Dallas, Dallas,
Texas

BRENDA BLAIN, DNP, RN, FACHE, NEA-BC
Baylor Medical Center at Irving, Irving, Texas

MAE M. CENTENO, DNP, RN, CCNS, ACNS-BC
Corporate Director, Chronic Care Continuum, Institute of Chronic Disease and Care
Redesign, Baylor Health Care System at Dallas, Dallas, Texas

CAROL CRENSHAW, MBA, BSN, RN
Clinical Manager, Baylor University Medical Center at Dallas, Dallas, Texas

SONYA A. FLANDERS, MSN, RN, ACNS-BC, CCRN
Clinical Nurse Specialist, Center for Learning Innovation and Practice, Baylor Scott & White Health, North Texas, Dallas, Texas

RITA J. FOWLER, MSN, RN, CCRN, NE-BC
Vice President, Critical Care Services, Department of Critical Care, Baylor University Medical Center at Dallas, Dallas, Texas

PAMELA GREEN, MSN, RN, FNP-BC
Department of Supportive and Palliative Care, Baylor Regional Medical Center at Carrollton, Carrollton, Texas

SHARON GUNN, MSN, MA, RN, ACNS-BC, CCRN
Clinical Nurse Specialist, Center for Learning Innovation and Practice, Baylor Health Care System at Dallas, Dallas, Texas

MARYGRACE HERNANDEZ-LEVEILLE, PhD, RN, ACNP-BC
Baylor University Medical Center at Dallas, Dallas, Texas

PENNY HUDDLESTON, PhD(c), RN, CCRN
Stroke Coordinator, Department of Administration, Baylor Medical Center at Irving, Irving, Texas

KELLIE L. KAHVECI, MSN, RN, AGPCNP-BC, GNP-BC, CHFN
Nurse Practitioner Manager, Baylor HouseCalls and Transitional Care Program, Health Texas Provider Network, Dallas, Texas

CAY KUBIN, BSN, RN, CNML
Manager, Intensive Care Unit, Baylor Medical Center at Waxahachie, Waxahachie, Texas

BARBARA LEEPER, MN, RN-BC, CNS M-S, CCRN, FAHA
Clinical Nurse Specialist, Cardiovascular Services, Baylor University Medical Center at Dallas, Dallas, Texas

DONNA MOREHEAD, MSN/INF, RN, NE-BC
Baylor Medical Center at Irving, Irving, Texas

CINDY MURRAY, MBA, MHA, BSN, RN, CENP, CNOR
Chief Nursing Officer/Chief Operating Officer, Department of Administration, Baylor Medical Center at Waxahachie, Waxahachie, Texas

NICOLE NELSON, MSN, RN, ACNP-BC, CCRN
Dallas Pulmonary & Critical Care PA, Dallas, Texas

ELIZABETH ORTIZ, MBA, BSN, RN, NEA-BC
Director, Acute Care Services; Nursing Administration, Baylor Medical Center at Waxahachie, Waxahachie, Texas

KRISTINE K. POWELL, MSN, RN, CEN, NEA-BC
Director of Emergency Services, Office of the Chief Nursing Officer, Baylor Scott & White–North Texas, Dallas, Texas

JAME RESTAU, MSN, RN, ACNS-BC, ACHPN
Department of Supportive and Palliative Care, Baylor Medical Center at Irving, Irving, Texas

KATHLEEN M. SHUEY, MS, RN, AOCN, ACNS-BC
Clinical Nurse Specialist, Department of Nursing, Oncology, Baylor University Medical Center, T. Boone Pickens Cancer Hospital, Dallas, Texas

LAUREN E. SMITH, BSN, RN, CCRN-CSC
Nurse Educator, Cardiothoracic & Heart-Lung Transplant ICU, Baylor University Medical Center at Dallas, Dallas, Texas

SUSAN SMITH, DNP, RN, ACNS-BC
Adult Clinical Nurse Specialist, Department of Critical Care Services, Baylor University Medical Center at Dallas, Dallas, Texas

TABITHA SOUTH, MSN, RN
Director of Critical Care and Nursing Administration, Baylor Regional Medical Center at Grapevine, Grapevine, Texas; Director, Medical Surgical Services, Medical Center of Plano, Plano, Texas

JESSICA H. STRASEN, BSN, RN, CCRN
Nurse Educator, 4 Truett Medical ICU, Baylor University Medical Center at Dallas, Dallas, Texas

EMYLENE UNTALAN, MSN, RN, CCRN, CPAN
Nurse Manager, Post Anesthesia Care Unit, Baylor University Medical Center at Dallas, Dallas, Texas

AMY VEENSTRA, RN, CCRN, CMC
Nursing Administrative Supervisor/Rapid Response Team Supervisor, Department of Nursing Administration, Baylor University Medical Center at Dallas, Dallas, Texas

MEGAN WHEELER, MSN, RN, ACNS-BC
Clinical Nurse Specialist, Baylor Health Care System at Dallas, Dallas, Texas

MARY BETH ZIMMERMANN, MSN, RN, ACNS-BC
Stroke Advanced Practice Nurse, Department of Stroke Administration, Texas Health Harris Methodist Fort Worth, Fort Worth, Texas

Contents

The global population is aging, and with that comes new challenges. Optimal care must be delivered to minimize the time spent in the acute care setting. Avoiding costly complications and focusing on health promotion rather than disease management will be key. Geriatrics is a complex patient population and basic nursing care is essential to prevent unnecessary complications if our health care system is to survive. Our profession is ill prepared to optimally care for this patient population.

This article discusses the history of the Comprehensive Unit-based Safety Program (CUSP) and how it is used to foster a culture of safety. CUSP involves interdisciplinary teamwork and empowers nurses at all levels to pioneer changes and develop leadership skills. A case study is presented to show how CUSP was used effectively in critical care to create a standardized handover of patients from the operating room to the intensive care unit.

Delirium in the intensive care unit is prevalent and a topic of high interest. Although it has been studied a great deal, screening, prevention, and management remain difficult. There are many causes of delirium and equally as many approaches to prevention and treatment. Two case studies sharing the challenges and successes of education, prevention, and treatment of delirium are presented in the context of complex adaptive systems.

Stroke is the fourth leading cause of death in the United States. On average, someone has a stroke every 40 seconds. The gaps for patients diagnosed with a stroke are the availability of physicians who specialize in stroke care and access to evidence-based stroke care. Telemedicine has assisted in bridging this gap to provide effective stroke treatment. The purpose of this article is to describe how the implementation of a hub and spoke model using telemedicine has assisted in increasing patient access to neurology expertise and receiving evidence-based treatment of

CRITICAL CARE NURSING
CLINICS OF NORTH AMERICA

Preface
Quality

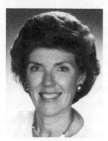 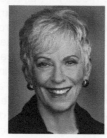

Barbara Leeper, MN, RN-BC, CNS   Rosemary Luquire, RN, PhD,
      M-S, CCRN, FAHA   NEA-BC, FAAN
                        Editors

This issue contains a series of articles focused on various initiatives aimed at improving the quality of patient care delivery and promoting safe passage across the continuum of care. Exemplary, evidence-based nursing practice is the cornerstone of quality care, and this issue highlights many ways in which nurses have led changes to optimize patient outcomes. In addition, quality care enhances cost-effectiveness by reducing avoidable complications and diminishing avoidable hospital readmissions, a concept more important than ever due to value-based purchasing and the Affordable Care Act.

Gunn and Fowler start the issue reminding us that the global population is aging and we, as a nursing community, are ill-prepared to provide safe care for these patients. They provide a review of the most vulnerable aspects of the older patient, followed by a case presentation exemplifying important points.

Handoff communication between clinicians is extremely important. Smith and Flanders describe a staff nurse–driven project implemented as part of the Comprehensive Unit-Based Safety Program in a cardiothoracic surgery intensive care unit (ICU). ICU staff nurses identified an opportunity to improve the patient handoff they received from anesthesia providers immediately on arrival of postcardiac surgery patients to the ICU. Through collaboration between anesthesiology and the nursing staff, a process titled the "Royal Exchange" was developed. The Royal Exchange facilitates transition of care from the operating room to the ICU and has been associated with improvements in blood glucose management, consistency in vasoactive and inotropic infusions, and communication about the myocardial status.

Several authors share examples of promoting safe passage of patients through the implementation of processes to assure evidence-based practices are hard-wired

Crit Care Nurs Clin N Am 26 (2014) xiii–xv
http://dx.doi.org/10.1016/j.cnc.2014.08.001
0899-5885/14/$ – see front matter © 2014 Published by Elsevier Inc.

across care settings. Wheeler and colleagues discuss delirium screening and prevention at a major health system by presenting two case studies, addressing the challenges and successes of education, prevention, and treatment of delirium in the context of complex adaptive systems. Huddleston and Zimmerman describe the success of a hub-and-spoke model for management of acute stroke patients within a large health care system. This model is exemplified by the subsequent article by Murray and colleagues describing the use of a robot for rounding in a small rural hospital. Powell and Fowler discuss the development of a partnership between the ICU and emergency department aimed at driving sepsis mortality down in a large urban medical center. Veenstra and Untalan discuss interventions implemented by a multidisciplinary team to protect patients with sleep apnea from oversedation and reduce patients' risk of respiratory arrest. Blain and colleagues reveal the strategies they used to drive their hospital-acquired pressure ulcers down to zero. Beseda and colleagues provide an overview of the complexity of therapeutic hypothermia, using a case study throughout their article. Shuey and colleagues discusses the importance of implementing a comprehensive fall prevention program with particular emphasis on the oncology patient population.

In recent years, the importance of family presence in the ICU has been recognized. South and Adair address current findings regarding the transition to open access and approaches taken by various units, hospitals, and health care systems to change the longstanding critical care culture. Next, Flanders and Strassen present relevant research on attitudes about family presence during resuscitation (FPDR), interventions to help change practice, and one medical ICU's experience with implementing FPDR. Restau and Green discuss how the integration of palliative care into the ICU provides care, comfort, and planning for patients, families, and the medical staff and helps decrease the emotional, spiritual, and psychological stress of a patient's death. They outline quality measures for palliative care in the ICU and use case studies to demonstrate how this integration can be beneficial for a patient and family.

The last three articles in this issue present strategies that can be used to address specific patient populations. Allen and Leeper review management of cardiogenic shock with an emphasis on extracorporeal membrane oxygenation (ECMO) and include a discussion of things to consider when determining who will run the ECMO circuit (perfusion vs nursing). Centeno and Kahveci share their experience within a large metropolitan health care system working to decrease readmission rates for an at-risk, geriatric patient population by utilizing a transitional care program. In the last article, Leveille and colleagues offer an overview of the role of an acute care nurse practitioner (ACNP) in the acute setting caring for patients with cardiovascular issues. They discuss the evolution of the role of the ACNP, and the Consensus Model for APRN regulation, and presents a case study highlighting the ACNP as a liaison between the patient, family members, collaborating physicians, and nurses.

It is our hope that you, the reader, are able to take a few of the lessons learned and experience the successes shared by the authors of the articles in this issue of *Critical Care Nursing Clinics of North America*.

Barbara Leeper, MN, RN-BC, CNS M-S, CCRN, FAHA
Cardiovascular Services
Baylor University Medical Center at Dallas
3500 Gaston Avenue
Truett Building, Suite 145
Dallas, TX 75246, USA

Rosemary Luquire, RN, PhD, NEA-BC, FAAN
Baylor Scott and White Health
North Texas
3600 Gaston Avenue
Wadley Tower, Suite 150
Dallas, TX 75246, USA

E-mail addresses:
bobbil@BaylorHealth.edu (B. Leeper)
RosemarL@BaylorHealth.edu (R. Luquire)

Back to Basics

Importance of Nursing Interventions in the Elderly Critical Care Patient

Sharon Gunn, MSN, MA, RN, ACNS-BC, CCRN[a],*,
Rita J. Fowler, MSN, RN, CCRN, NE-BC[b]

KEYWORDS

• Geriatrics • Health care • Complexity • Chronic conditions • Nursing

KEY POINTS

• Older adults are a complex patient population.
• The nursing workforce is ill prepared to provide optimal care for this population.
• A "back to basics" approach to nursing care can help to prevent unnecessary complications during hospitalization.
• A knowledge of geriatrics, the ability to adapt care to individual patients, and interdisciplinary teamwork and communication are essential across all transitions of care.

The world's population is aging, and global predictions estimate that the largest growth sector from 2013 to 2050 will be persons over 60 years of age. By year 2030, 1 in every 8 persons on the planet will be over the age of 65.[1] The United Nations predicts that this sector of the world's population will triple by the year 2100, reaching 27% of the total global population.[2] The reasons for this are 3-fold: People are living longer healthier lives, there are global declines in fertility, and baby boomers are reaching retirement.[3,4] The situation is similar in the United States, with population increases of persons over 65 years expected to more than double from 2010 to 2050 (Fig. 1).[5] As population demographics shift, in future decades we will also see a rise in noncommunicable disease that has the potential to stretch our already burdened health care system beyond its limits.[3] Persons with chronic conditions such as heart failure, obesity, chronic obstructive pulmonary disease (COPD), hypertension, and more, consume vast amounts of our health care resources.[6,7] Alzheimer disease is the sixth leading cause of death in the United States.[8] Today, an American is

The authors have nothing to disclose.
[a] Center for Learning Innovation and Practice, Baylor Health Care System at Dallas, 2001 Bryan Street, Suite 601, Dallas, TX 75201, USA; [b] Critical Care Services, Baylor University Medical Center at Dallas, 3500 Gaston Avenue, Dallas, TX 75246, USA
* Corresponding author.
E-mail address: Sharon.gunn@baylorhealth.edu

Crit Care Nurs Clin N Am 26 (2014) 433–446
http://dx.doi.org/10.1016/j.ccell.2014.08.012
0899-5885/14/$ – see front matter © 2014 Elsevier Inc. All rights reserved.

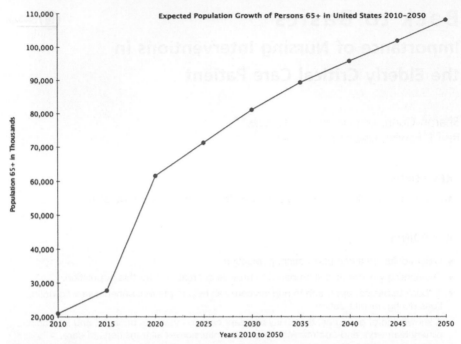

Fig. 1. Projected U.S. population increase for persons over 65. (*Data from* US Census Bureau. 2008 National population projections: summary tables. Projections of the population by selected age groups and sex for the United States: 2010 to 2050. Available at: http://www. census.gov/population/projections/data/national/2008/summarytables.html. Accessed August 8, 2014.)

diagnosed with Alzheimer disease every 68 seconds, and by 2050 this diagnosis will occur every 33 seconds.[8]

The workforce is ill prepared to care for an aging demographic: Health care professionals traditionally have little or no curricular content dedicated to geriatric care.[9] Over half the patients hospitalized in the United States are over 65 years old, but less than 1% of the current nursing workforce is certified in geriatrics.[10]

Most of us who have been in practice for many years have traditionally "clumped" the geriatric patient population with young and middle-aged adults. As critical care nurses, we know that our practice is a specialized area, and that specific skills, critical thinking, and prioritization are vital to provide the best care possible for our patients. Most of us would not hesitate to admit our lack of expertise in, for example, pediatrics. If we were in a position where we were outside of our area of expertise we would seek help, information, and perhaps pursue educational offerings to build a sound knowledge base.

Many nursing professionals may not realize the extent to which the geriatric population consumes health care resources, or the complexity in care that older adults bring to the table. From a cost perspective, in 2013 the annual cost of Alzheimer disease to the United States was $203 billion, and by 2050 this cost is projected to reach $1.2 trillion annually.[8] Cardiovascular disease and diabetes alone cost the United States over $750 billion every year.[11] One in 5 elderly adults are readmitted to the hospital within 30 days of discharge.[12] Not only are hospital readmissions costly in terms of finance, but also in terms of morbidity, mortality, and reduced quality of life. Most hospital readmissions are unplanned and have been associated with poor discharge planning, poor coordination of care, and ineffective communication of health care workers with each other, patients, and their families.[12,13]

So what do we need to do to provide patient-centered, quality care to our geriatric patient population? Five areas are addressed herein where astute critical care nurses can really make a difference in patient outcomes: The aging body, resiliency and vulnerability, functional status, polypharmacy, and chronic conditions. An overview of the complexity of older adult care in the intensive care unit (ICU) will follow a case study to help clarify and illustrate how nursing can make a difference in geriatric patient outcomes.

THE AGING BODY

The majority of older Americans consider themselves to be in good or excellent health (**Fig. 2**).[14] Many remain active and independent well into their latter decades. Changes occur in our body systems as we age, and although daily functioning is maintained, the result of these age-related changes is that older adults have less reserve to bounce back from a health-related insult. Decreased reserve along with normal age-related changes makes us more vulnerable to complications or interactions with medications. What is important to note is that older adults often present to the acute care facility with atypical signs and symptoms of disease.[15] Atypical presentation of disease in addition to increased vulnerability for complications is 1 reason why an understanding of normal, age-related changes is necessary. We must know what is normal to differentiate normal age-related changes from pathologic conditions.

Using a head-to-toe concise approach, some of the basics of age-related changes are presented herein. There is variability among individuals in the way we age, making individualized care more challenging for the astute critical care nurse.[16]

In the neurologic system, we have a decreasing number of functional neurons as we age, and transmission of information slows.[17] This results in more time needed to learn and process new information, which has implications for meticulous and ongoing

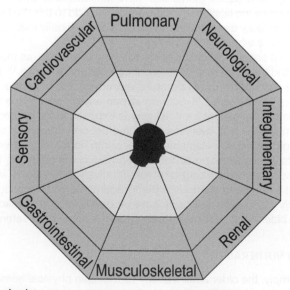

Fig. 2. The aging body.

patient education. The hypothalamus does not regulate temperature as effectively, so atypical presentation of conditions, like pneumonia and sepsis, may occur. Proprioception decreases, as does our ability to adapt to changes in position, making falls more likely.[17] The senses dull, and eyesight, hearing, touch, taste, and smell are less acute. A decreased ability to smell and taste can negatively affect appetite in an elderly individual who is ill. Decreased visual acuity may increase risk for falls in an unfamiliar environment.

The cardiopulmonary system is less efficient, resulting in decreased cardiac output, decreased ability to increase heart rate in response to stress, and overall decreased blood flow systemically.[18] Older adults adapt to these changes quite well until increased or unusual demands are placed on the body: Perhaps they have to take the stairs when the elevator is broken or rush to cross a street before the traffic light changes to green. Increased peripheral resistance results in an increased systolic blood pressure. There are fewer alveoli in the lungs and decreased elasticity owing to calcification of the costal cartilage.[18] The cough reflex is diminished, as is the ability to clear secretions.[18] These and other changes lead to lower exercise tolerance and gas exchange, and increased susceptibility to pneumonia. Add to this the real possibility that the older patient you may see will most likely have comorbid conditions such as COPD or heart failure, taxing these body systems further.

The entire gastrointestinal system is affected by aging, and is often more bothersome than life threatening. Lesser saliva production, decreased number of taste buds, and decreased ability to digest starch and tolerate fats, make indigestion and constipation more likely.[17] Absorption of nutrients, vitamins and minerals is less efficient, particularly calcium and vitamin D, which are important in prevention of osteoporosis and other illnesses. Hepatic laboratory tests tend to remain normal, but hepatic enzymes decrease in number and the liver is less efficient at metabolizing and excreting toxins. This makes drug toxicities more likely. The renal system also becomes less effective: Between the ages of 20 and 90, renal blood flow and glomerular filtration rate decrease by 50% or more.[18] Older kidneys are less able to conserve sodium and utilize antidiuretic hormone, making both hyponatremia and dehydration a distinct possibility. Decreased glomerular filtration rate and decreased creatinine clearance can increase the likelihood for drug toxicity. Add to this the fact that persons over 65 are the most likely demographic to be on 5 or more daily medications, and polypharmacy takes on a whole new meaning.

Perhaps the most observable changes are thinning of the skin, as the subcutaneous fat layer is lost, and the epidermis thins and becomes more fragile.[18] This makes the older adult more susceptible to temperature extremes, and hyperthermia and hypothermia are distinct possibilities. Hypothermia can easily occur in the hospital during bathing, particularly if the patient's entire body is exposed in the process. The musculoskeletal system stiffens and weakens. Muscles become atrophied and flabby, and joints become rigid and stiff.[16] Gait changes occur in both men and women. Regular exercise helps to minimize some of these negative consequences, but placing an older adult on bed rest can have long-term ramifications on functional status and quality of life. Normal age-related changes in the integumentary and musculoskeletal system automatically place older adults at increased risk for skin breakdown and falls, even before the older adult becomes a patient in the acute care setting.

RESILIENCY AND VULNERABILITY

To put it quite simply, the older adult's ability to maintain physical homeostasis is less robust than younger adults (**Fig. 3**).[19] A 20-year-old admitted to the hospital with

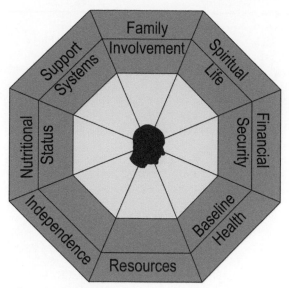

Fig. 3. Factors contributing to resiliency and vulnerability.

community-acquired pneumonia is much more likely to bounce back to full recovery than an older adult. Pneumonia in a geriatric patient can be devastating, particularly if there are underlying conditions such as COPD or heart failure. Under these circumstances, the older adult's resilience is diminished. But resilience is not only about dealing with changes in physical health. Other factors play into the equation, such as lifestyle habits, social support, spiritual beliefs, and the ability to deal with adversity.[20] As we age, we are more likely to encounter loss of friends, loved ones, and independence. All of these factors play a part in our ability to deal with illness and bounce back to baseline health.

The older adult is more vulnerable to hospital-acquired conditions, such as pressure ulcers, falls, and delirium. Physiologic changes that occur with aging partially contribute to this increased risk, but the acute care environment and care we provide also plays a significant role. Immobility, prolonged bed rest, lack of sleep, and an unfamiliar environment are a few of the elements introduced that contribute to the likelihood something may go wrong.

The incidence of delirium in older adult patients has been reported to be as high as 87% in some studies, and is an independent risk factor for increased morbidity, mortality, duration of stay, and long-term cognitive decline.[21–23] The critical care nurse must not only know how to prevent or minimize the onset of delirium in the older adult, but must also have the knowledge to identify delirium in persons who may also have an underlying depression or dementia.[24]

FUNCTIONAL STATUS

Functional status refers to our ability to perform independent activities of daily living, activities of daily living, and maintain independence and quality of life (**Fig. 4**). Hospital admission can be a significant cause of functional decline in persons older than 65, and affects anywhere from 30% to 60% or more of inpatients.[25–28] Functional decline has been reported to occur by day 2 of hospitalization, and has devastating

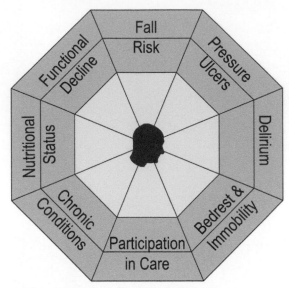

Fig. 4. Complexity of functional status in older adults.

consequences, such as increased mortality, morbidity, duration of stay, long-term care placement, and hospital readmissions.[29,30] Many patients never regain full prehospitalization function.[31] Although preexisting patient conditions and the disease processes play a part in functional decline in the hospital, iatrogenic causes such as immobility and bed rest are mostly to blame.[30,32]

Ideally, older adults who are admitted to the hospital would not suffer functional decline. Mobility, balance, and gait assessment and training in addition to adequate nutrition during hospitalization should be the norm rather than the exception. At the very least, ICU patients should receive frequent range of motion and repositioning in bed. If able, sitting in a chair for all meals and ambulation should occur daily.

POLYPHARMACY

Polypharmacy is an alarming phenomenon in caring for persons over the age of 65 (**Fig. 5**). It increases the complexity of care, and risks for adverse events to occur. Polypharmacy not only refers to the number of medications a person takes on a daily basis, but includes the following factors: Multiple prescribers, different pharmacies dispensing medications, inappropriate use of medications that have no clinical indication for use, multiple dosing schedules, drugs in the same family of medication being prescribed for different conditions, prescriptions that are continued long after the condition has subsided, and use of over-the-counter and herbal remedies.[33]

Polypharmacy is more than an issue of multiple medications. We have already mentioned changes in the body as we age. These age-related changes affect pharmacokinetics and pharmacodynamics.[34] Pharmacokinetics results in changes in absorption, distribution, metabolism, and excretion of medications. Pharmacodynamics is how the drug affects the patient. The American Geriatrics Society developed the Beers criteria to identify potentially inappropriate medications for use older adults owing to the increased incidence of adverse drug events.[35] Although this is certainly a useful tool, it does not address guidelines on combinations of medications that frequently

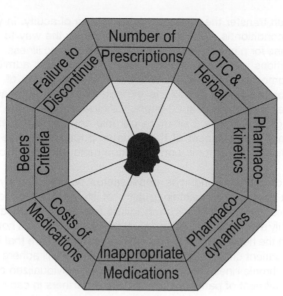

Fig. 5. Elements of polypharmacy in older adults.

occur in older adults with multiple comorbid conditions.[36] Moreover, when hospitalized, older adults are frequently prescribed new medications to treat the acute illness. Inappropriate use of medications, and failure to perform a thorough medication reconciliation before and after transitions in care, have resulted in increased morbidity (falls, decreased functional status, and delirium), mortality, and rehospitalization.[36]

CHRONIC CONDITIONS

Patients admitted to the ICU are usually there because of an acute illness, or exacerbation of a preexisting condition (**Fig. 6**). We are focused on "fixing" the acute

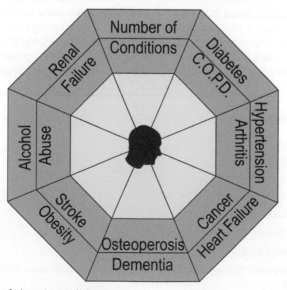

Fig. 6. Examples of chronic conditions.

problem, and then transfer the patient to a lower area of acuity. In younger adults, once the acute condition is resolved, they are often on the way to a full recovery. This is not the case for persons who have to live with chronic illness. The prevalence of chronic conditions increases with age, and often patients admitted to the ICU have multiple comorbid conditions, and consume the majority of health care resources.[6] Noncommunicable disease is expected to place increased burden on health care systems over the next 30 years.[37] Anywhere from 50% to 80% of persons over the age of 65 have 1 or more chronic conditions.[18] What adds to the complexity of care in this subset of the geriatric population is the fact that often treatment guidelines for 1 chronic condition contradict treatment for other chronic conditions.[38,39]

Management of chronic conditions necessitates participation by the patient to follow treatment plans, and maintain quality of life and independence.[40] Poorly managed diabetes, hypertension, or heart failure may result in repeated hospitalizations for potentially avoidable situations. Many times, the patient is not to blame. Success depends on the health care team developing a plan of care that will work for the patient, that the patient understands, and that the patient will adhere to.[41,42] Optimal management of chronic illness begins in the ICU with individualized care, patient education, and recruitment of patients and families as partners in care.

CASE STUDY

Mrs Campbell is an 87-year-old, frail lady who is admitted to the ICU with a diagnosis of community-acquired pneumonia. She has a history of heart failure, COPD, rheumatoid arthritis, hypertension, and osteoporosis. She had an aortic valve replacement 10 years ago and has not had any complications from the surgery. She is widowed and lives alone, but is very active in her church and manages to care for herself independently. She has a son who lives in the same city as she does. She is well educated, and lives on a limited budget owing to her monthly medication bills to manage her chronic conditions. Her medication regimen is presented in **Box 1**.

Mrs Campbell has successfully managed her chronic illnesses for many years, and has been hospitalized twice in the past 2 years for community-acquired pneumonia. Other history includes a 50 pack-year smoker (she quit smoking 20 years ago), walks around her neighborhood block twice a day, and eating a heart-healthy diet. Two days before admission, Mrs Campbell had been feeling weak with increased shortness of breath on exertion. She had been extremely nauseated, with diarrhea, and had little

---

Box 1
Mrs Campbell's medications

Methotrexate 75 mg once a week

Coreg 6.25 mg twice a day

Lisinopril 10 mg once a day

Furosemide 20 mg twice a day

Advair 250 mcg twice a day

Coumadin 5 mg Monday, Wednesday, and Friday

Centrum Silver and a potassium supplement once a day

Hydrocodone 5 mg/APAP 325 mg every 6 hours as needed for pain related to rheumatoid arthritis flare-ups

to eat or drink. Her son brought her some extra-strength Tylenol and Imodium AD from the grocery store to help her combat her symptoms.

Mrs Campbell is admitted to your unit via the emergency department (ED). In the ED she was worked up for sepsis: Laboratory studies, chest x-ray, and blood gasses were obtained. She received 2 L of normal saline, and her first dose of antibiotics. A Foley catheter and central line were also placed in the ED.

On admission to the ICU, she is restless with marked work of breathing. She is acutely delirious, pulling at her oxygen mask, and insisting she get out of bed to go to the bathroom. Her O_2 saturation is 91% on 100% nonrebreather mask. Blood pressure is 108/86 mm Hg, rapid atrial fibrillation is present, respiratory rate is 32, and she is afebrile. The decision is made to intubate, and Mrs Campbell is placed on mechanical ventilation using assist-control, pressure support, and positive end-expiratory pressure. She is also placed on a propofol drip for sedation and in-line nebulizer treatments are initiated. Her initial laboratory workup indicates that she is positive for sepsis. Her lactate level is 2.6, and she is severely dehydrated. She is in acute renal failure, and her liver enzymes are slightly elevated.

Scheduled intravenous doses of levaquin are initiated to treat her pneumonia. She receives 2 more liters of saline bolus followed by a continuous IV drip.

Over the course of the next several days, Mrs Campbell's pneumonia is resolving and she successfully weans from the ventilator. She transfers out of the ICU on day 4. Although you may consider the care you provided routine basic nursing care, it was, in fact, life saving.

BACK TO BASICS

The importance of basic nursing care for Mrs Campbell's safety cannot be overemphasized. The first thing to note is that Mrs Campbell has multiple chronic conditions. A COPD exacerbation, or in this case a pneumonia, can really set back her ability to keep mobile and active. Mobility equals independence in Mrs Campbell's situation. Loss of mobility leads to loss of function and muscle atrophy. As soon as is possibly feasible, Mrs Campbell must get up out of bed and ambulate. At the very least, passive range of motion and a physical therapy consult should be initiated on admission. Keeping Mrs Campbell on bed rest affects every body system, but the difference between a 20-year-old and an 87-year-old, is that bed rest could place Mrs Campbell in a position where she does not have the physical ability to recover to a prehospitalized state of health.

Mobility is also important in preventing hospital-acquired pressure ulcers. On your admission assessment, Mrs Campbell already has a stage 1 pressure ulcer on her sacrum and her spine between the scapula. She has only been in the facility a few short hours. Her age, frailty, and now immobility place her at high risk. As her nurse, extra vigilance is required to keep Mrs Campbell's skin intact.

Next, we must look at polypharmacy. Polypharmacy is common in adults over 65 years of age, particularly if they have 2 or more chronic conditions.[43] Mrs Campbell has been successfully managing her conditions for years, but there are a couple of "alarms" that go off right away. The over-the-counter medications her son brought her may have adverse effects on her condition. She is now receiving additional medications as an inpatient. Medication reconciliation is a priority across care transitions, which is where most medication discrepancies occur. Medication discrepancies are costly in terms of morbidity, increased duration of stay, and costs.[44]

Accurate inputs and outputs will be necessary to ensure adequate hydration and resolution of her acute renal failure. Her renal system is already compromised owing to her age and current physiologic condition, but electrolyte imbalance is a real possibility, and with her history of heart failure, you must keep on top of all of these factors to prevent lethal arrhythmias. Nutrition is also included in this category and will play a vital role in Mrs Campbell's healing. She is elderly, so her taste and olfactory sensations are likely diminished. She is not feeling well, so it may be challenging to get her to receive enough nutrients after extubation.

Good sleep hygiene and frequent reorientation to her surroundings will be paramount for healing, but also to resolve her acute delirious state as quickly as possible. The longer she is delirious, the worse her outcomes will be in terms of cognitive decline, morbidity, mortality, duration of stay, and long-term care placement. You encourage her son and other family members to bring in familiar objects or photographs, keep the lights on during the day, and dim them at night. During daylight hours, have her sit up on the side of the bed or in the chair, and ambulate as her condition warrants, so that she is tired and pharmacologic assistance for sleep is avoided. You make sure Mrs Campbell is not restrained, and as she improves daily rounding with the physicians will involve discussion of the need for lines, tubes, or drains.

Even after 1 day in bed, Mrs Campbell is deconditioned. Your priority will be to get her up out of bed with assistance to ambulate. Failure to do so will not only promote functional decline and threaten future independence, but it will also increase her fall risk should she become any more deconditioned.

Patient and family education and involvement in care are essential. You are fortunate that Mrs Campbell is quite active and able to manage her chronic conditions. Many persons either cannot or will not participate in self-care. This is particularly challenging with chronic conditions, where compliance with diet, medication regimens, and physician visits often means the difference between a hospital visit or normal daily life.

COMPLEXITY AND CARE OF THE OLDER ADULT

Hopefully by now you will have realized that there is more to caring for the older adult than medically managing their diagnosis (**Fig. 7**). We have merely touched the surface of how complex geriatric care is. Each person ages differently, and has a unique health history and lifestyle choices. Each individual may or may not be capable of managing their own health maintenance, chronic illness, or have the social and financial support required to purchase medications, make doctors' appointments, and follow multiple health-related instructions. Each basic element that forms the building blocks of a person's life must be considered to provide the best care possible for that patient on any given day.

Whether you have heard of complexity science or not, it is hard to deny that the health care environment is increasing in complexity. Within the ICU there are multiple disciplines and departments working to get the job done. Nursing takes care of patients, families, equipment, coordinating care, and documentation in the medical record. Each element of the system works interdependently to organize and produce sometimes unpredictable, and often unexpected, outcomes. Sometimes a day in the ICU seems totally chaotic, but everything seems to work out just fine. This is the essence of a complex adaptive system.[45] Complex adaptive systems contain some core elements: Multiple components, interactivity, emergence, and feedback.[46] To work successfully in such an environment, nurses must be fluid enough to adapt to changing conditions, deal with unexpected outcomes in real time, and understand that different combinations of disease, treatments, and responses do not yield identical outcomes.

Geriatric nursing demands adaptability, knowledge of the unique challenges facing this population, and the ability to competently care for every individual encountered.

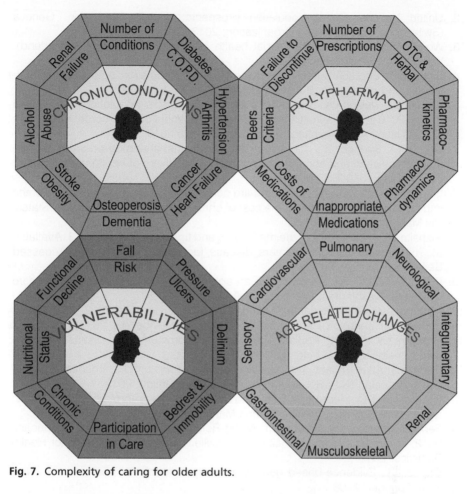

Fig. 7. Complexity of caring for older adults.

The combination of multiple chronic diseases is treated differently than one alone. Multiple medications interact together differently than each one alone. Each patient's lifestyle, culture, willingness to participate in care, and ability to finance needed treatments are some of the elements that must be taken into consideration if our health care system is to adapt to challenges ahead.

We have glimpsed some of the components of nursing care of the geriatric patient. Future success depends on our ability to communicate and function as true interdisciplinary teams, across all care transitions. We will learn to manage chronic disease outside of the acute care setting. Focus will be placed on disease prevention and health promotion. Patient and family involvement with the health care team will be integral and essential. We must adapt to these current challenges, and change the way health care is delivered so that we can be successful in meeting the needs of the aging population ahead.

REFERENCES

1. National Institute on Aging. Why population aging matters: a global perspective. Bethesda (MD): National Institute on Aging; 2007.

2. United Nations. World population prospects: the 2012 revision. Geneva (Switzerland): World Health Organization; 2013.
3. World Health Organization. Global health and ageing. Geneva (Switzerland): World Health Organization; 2011.
4. Bloom DE, Boersch-Supan A, McGee P, et al. Population aging: facts, challenges, and responses. Benefit Compensat Int 2011;41(1):22.
5. Vincent GK, Velkoff VA. The next four decades: the older population in the United States: 2010 to 2050. Washington, DC: US Department of Commerce, Economics and Statistics Administration, US Census Bureau; 2010.
6. Denton FT, Spencer BG. Chronic health conditions: changing prevalence in an aging population and some implications for the delivery of health care services. Can J Aging 2010;29(01):11–21.
7. Garrett N, Martini EM. The boomers are coming: a total cost of care model of the impact of population aging on the cost of chronic conditions in the United States. Dis Manag 2007;10(2):51–60.
8. Alzheimer's Association. Alzheimer's facts and figures. Updated 2013. Available at: http://www.alz.org/alzheimers_disease_facts_and_figures.asp. Accessed September 18, 2013.
9. Institute of Medicine. Retooling for an aging America: building the health care workforce. Washington, DC: Institute of Medicine; 2008.
10. Hartford Institute for Geriatric Nursing. Certification. Updated 2012. Available at: http://consultgerirn.org/certification. Accessed September 18, 2013.
11. Narayan KV, Ali MK, Koplan JP. Global noncommunicable diseases—where worlds meet. N Engl J Med 2010;363(13):1196–8.
12. Dartmouth Atlas Project. The revolving door: a report on U.S. hospital readmissions. Princeton (NJ): Robert Wood Johnson Foundation; 2013.
13. Coddington DC, Moore KD. Reducing healthcare costs through better chronic disease management. Healthc Financ Manage 2012;66(8):126–8.
14. Federal Interagency Forum on Aging-Related Statistics. Older Americans 2012: key indicators of well-being. Hyattsville (MD): National Center for Health Statistics; 2012.
15. Capezuti L. Evidence-based geriatric nursing protocols for best practice. New York: Springer; 2008.
16. Brock AJ, Jablonski RA. Physiology of aging: impact on critical illness and treatment. In: Foreman MD, Milisen K, Fulmer TT, editors. Critical care nursing of older adults: best practices. 3rd edition. New York: Springer; 2010. p. 241–66.
17. Brown JB, Bedford NK, White SJ. Gerontological protocols for nurse practitioners. Philadelphia: Lippincott; 1999.
18. Eliopoulos C. Gerontological nursing. Philadelphia: Wolters Kluwer Health; 2013.
19. Clark PG, Burbank PM, Greene G, et al. What do we know about resilience in older adults? an exploration of some facts, factors, and facets. In: Resnick B, Gwyther LP, Roberto K, editors. Resilience in aging: concepts, research, and outcomes. New York: Springer; 2011. p. 51–66.
20. Hildon Z, Montgomery SM, Blane D, et al. Examining resilience of quality of life in the face of health-related and psychosocial adversity at older ages: what is "right" about the way we age? Gerontologist 2010;50(1):36–47.
21. Ouimet S, Kavanagh BP, Gottfried SB, et al. Incidence, risk factors and consequences of ICU delirium. Intensive Care Med 2007;33(1):66–73.
22. Pandharipande P, Shintani A, Peterson J, et al. Lorazepam is an independent risk factor for transitioning to delirium in intensive care unit patients. Anesthesiology 2006;104(1):21–6.

23. Inouye SK, Bogardus SJ, Baker DI, et al. The hospital elder life program: a model of care to prevent cognitive and functional decline in older hospitalized patients. J Am Geriatr Soc 2000;48(12):1697–706.
24. Foreman MD, Schuurmans M, Milisen K. Delirium in critical illness. In: Foreman MD, Milisen K, Fulmer TT, editors. Critical care nursing of older adults: best practices. 3rd edition. New York: Springer; 2010. p. 577–97.
25. Arora VM, Plein C, Chen S, et al. Relationship between quality of care and functional decline in hospitalized vulnerable elders. Med Care 2009;47(8): 895–901.
26. Black SA, Rush RD. Cognitive and functional decline in adults aged 75 and older. J Am Geriatr Soc 2002;50(12):1978–86.
27. Boltz M, Greenberg SA. Reducing functional decline in older adults during hospital-ization: a best practice approach. Try this: best practices in nursing care to older adults. New York: The Hartford Institute for Geriatric Nursing; 2012 (31). Available at: http://consultgerirn.org/uploads/File/trythis/try_this_31.pdf. Accessed October 25, 2012.
28. Braes T, Flamaing J, Sterckx W, et al. Predicting the risk of functional decline in older patients admitted to the hospital: a comparison of three screening instru-ments. Age Ageing 2009;38:600–22.
29. Graf C. Functional decline in hospitalized older adults: it's often a consequence of hospitalization, but it doesn't have to be. Am J Nurs 2006;106(1):58–68, 2p.
30. Hoogerduijn JG, Schuurmans MJ, Duijnstee MS, et al. A systematic review of pre-dictors and screening instruments to identify older hospitalized patients at risk for functional decline. J Clin Nurs 2006;16:46–57.
31. Sager MA, Franke T, Inouye SK, et al. Functional outcomes of acute medical illness and hospitalization in older persons. Arch Intern Med 1996;156(6):645.
32. Winkelman C. Bed rest in health and critical illness: a body systems approach. AACN Adv Crit Care 2009;20(3):254–66.
33. Planton J, Edlund BJ. Strategies for reducing polypharmacy in older adults. J Gerontol Nurs 2010;36(1):8–12.
34. Kaufman G. Polypharmacy in older adults. Nurs Stand 2011;25(38):49–55 [quiz: 58].
35. Fick D, Semla T, Beizer J, et al. American geriatrics society updated beers criteria for potentially inappropriate medication use in older adults. J Am Geriatr Soc 2012;60(4):616–31.
36. Hilmer S, Gnjidic D. The effects of polypharmacy in older adults. Clin Pharmacol Ther 2008;85(1):86–8.
37. Epping-Jordan J, Pruitt S, Bengoa R, et al. Improving the quality of health care for chronic conditions. Qual Health Care 2004;13(4):299–305.
38. Upshur RE, Tracy S. Chronicity and complexity is what's good for the diseases always good for the patients? Can Fam Physician 2008;54(12):1655–8.
39. Boyd CM, Darer J, Boult C, et al. Clinical practice guidelines and quality of care for older patients with multiple comorbid diseases. JAMA 2005;294(6):716–24.
40. De Geest S, Steeman E, Leventhal ME, et al. Complexity in caring for an ageing heart failure population: concomitant chronic conditions and age related impair-ments. Eur J Cardiovasc Nurs 2004;3(4):263–70.
41. Hendrix CC, Wojciechowski CW. Chronic care management for the elderly: an opportunity for gerontological nurse practitioners. J Am Acad Nurse Pract 2005;17(7):263–7.
42. Shippee ND, Shah ND, May CR, et al. Cumulative complexity: a functional, patient-centered model of patient complexity can improve research and practice. J Clin Epidemiol 2012;65(10):1041–51.

43. Loya AM, González-Stuart A, Rivera JO. Prevalence of polypharmacy, polyherbacy, nutritional supplement use and potential product interactions among older adults living on the United States-Mexico border: a descriptive, questionnaire-based study. Drugs Aging 2009;26(5):423–36.
44. Villanyi D, Fok M, Wong RY. Medication reconciliation: identifying medication discrepancies in acutely ill hospitalized older adults. Am J Geriatr Pharmacother 2011;9(5):339–44.
45. Chaffee MW, McNeill MM. A model of nursing as a complex adaptive system. Nurs Outlook 2007;55:232–41.
46. Clancy TR. Navigating in a complex nursing world. J Nurs Adm 2004;34(6): 274–82.

Application of a Comprehensive Unit-Based Safety Program in Critical Care

The Royal Exchange

Lauren E. Smith, BSN, RN, CCRN-CSC[a],*,
Sonya A. Flanders, MSN, RN, ACNS-BC, CCRN[b]

KEYWORDS

- Communication • Comprehensive Unit-based Safety Program • Patient safety
- Patient handovers • Patient handoffs • Teamwork

KEY POINTS

- The Comprehensive Unit-based Safety Program focuses on improving patient safety at the unit level by fostering a culture of safety and involving front-line clinicians.
- The Comprehensive Unit-based Safety Program has been used successfully to reduce health care–associated infections and improve the patient safety climate in many hospital units across the United States.
- Nurses at all levels have leadership roles in the Comprehensive Unit-based Safety Program, which draws upon bedside caregivers' wisdom to solve problems and improve processes.
- Postoperative handovers are a critical time for a complex, vulnerable patient population; a structured handover can help mitigate the potential for communication errors.

Patient safety gained national attention in 1999 when the Institute of Medicine reported staggering numbers of people were dying in hospitals as a result of preventable medical errors.[1] Since then, there has been a sharp focus within health care to improve patient safety. The public, accrediting bodies, regulatory agencies, health care organizations, and clinicians have engaged in a plethora of activities aimed at improving reliability of health care delivery to achieve quality outcomes and reduce errors. Aside from the obvious desire to provide safe patient care, public reporting of quality measures and changes in reimbursement have been important drivers for hospital leaders

---

Disclosure Statement: The authors have no significant relationships to disclose.
[a] Cardiothoracic & Heart-Lung Transplant ICU, Baylor University Medical Center at Dallas, 3500 Gaston Avenue, Dallas, TX 75246, USA; [b] Center for Learning Innovation and Practice, Baylor Scott and White Health, North Texas, Dallas, Texas, USA
* Corresponding author.
E-mail address: lauren.smith@baylorhealth.edu

Crit Care Nurs Clin N Am 26 (2014) 447–460
http://dx.doi.org/10.1016/j.ccell.2014.08.004
0899-5885/14/$ – see front matter © 2014 Elsevier Inc. All rights reserved.

and clinicians to take action. Experts suggest there has been progress in patient safety, but gaps remain.[2] This article discusses the history of the Comprehensive Unit-Based Safety Program (CUSP) and how CUSP is used to foster a culture of safety.

PATIENT SAFETY: ISSUES AND APPROACHES

Nurses are key stakeholders in provision of safe, quality patient care, both within their own scopes of practice and as members of the interdisciplinary health team. Each day nurses take deliberate steps to prevent avoidable adverse events including medication errors, health care–acquired infections, pressure ulcers, falls, and wrong-site procedures. Nurses involved in direct patient care have an integral role in keeping patients safe because they spend the most time with patients, see the big picture of patient care, and are the hub of communication with other health care team members. In fact, contemporary nursing practice has been described as a complex adaptive system.[3] Because of the complexities of nursing and health care, nurses at all levels need to be leaders.[3] Because of their expertise in patient care processes, bedside nurses are well poised to lead or contribute to patient safety efforts as long as supportive organizational structures and processes are in place.

A key element of support necessary to eliminate gaps in patient safety is a culture of safety. Features of a culture of safety include holding everyone accountable for following safe practices regardless of position or power gradients and blameless reporting of errors and risks to safety.[4] These features sound simple, but changing a culture is difficult and requires the unwavering dedication of hospital leaders to ensure team members trust they will be supported when acting in accordance with expected behaviors. Organizations with a solid culture of safety analyze errors and near misses to determine root causes, aim to mitigate future risks, and share these findings so others can learn from them. Understanding root causes of errors helps health care teams implement improvement activities specifically to address those causes.

As of yet, no single best way to improve patient safety has been identified, although many process improvement approaches aimed at achieving desirable quality and safety outcomes have been used in health care. For example, the Institute for Healthcare Improvement has led efforts at using bundles of evidence-based practices to improve patient outcomes.[5] The first bundle approach was tested in 2001, and now bundles are used in many hospitals to drive reliable patient care. For example, critical care nurses are generally familiar with the ventilator bundle promoted by the Institute for Healthcare Improvement.[6] Another tactic to standardize processes and diminish errors has been to use checklists, such as those produced by the World Health Organization.[7] Some recommend a combination of processes and tools to improve safety rather than a single approach. For example, leaders of the Joint Commission recently suggested hospitals implement Robust Process Improvement, which combines methods of change management, Lean, and Six Sigma.[8]

Many improvement methods enlist the team approach to enhance quality and safety. As such, some programs focus heavily on building stronger teams. One of these, TeamSTEPPS, is a curriculum led by the Agency for Healthcare Research and Quality (AHRQ) and the Department of Defense. TeamSTEPPS is geared toward improving teamwork skills to create a culture of safety.[9] Another model, the Comprehensive Unit-based Safety Program (CUSP), incorporates teamwork, communication and leadership to promote patient safety at the unit level by involving front-line staff.[10] The CUSP framework initially was used in 2001 to tackle catheter-related bloodstream infections (BSI) in intensive care units (ICUs).[11] Since CUSP's inception, the program has expanded considerably, receiving national support and attention. Critical care nurses interested in fostering a unit culture of safety and taking actions to improve patient safety might consider CUSP as an improvement framework.

COMPREHENSIVE UNIT-BASED SAFETY PROGRAM

A foundational premise of CUSP revolves around culture and recognition that culture varies by unit within a hospital.[12] This premise underpins the intention for CUSP to be implemented at the unit level. CUSP incorporates a team approach to change management which includes front-line staff, team leaders, and senior leaders.[13] The program was initially tested in 2001 at the Johns Hopkins Hospital as an 8-step process, first in one ICU with a second ICU acting as a control unit.[12,14] The first step was a culture of safety assessment, after which staff received specific safety education and identified concerns, senior executives became involved with units, improvements were implemented, results were analyzed and shared, and the culture was reassessed.[14] One value of CUSP is that successes arising from unit-based initiatives can be spread to other areas.[15] As such, CUSP was implemented in the second (control) ICU 6 months after the first unit had implemented the program.[14] Several improvements resulted, including creation of a daily goal sheet, which promoted communication and safety, and a defined medication reconciliation process when patients had orders to leave the ICU. A transport team and point-of-care pharmacist were funded as a result of staff concerns. Medication errors on transfer from the ICUs were eliminated, patient length of stay was shortened, and nursing turnover decreased. Follow-up assessment found more positive scores on the safety culture survey in both units, indicating the culture had indeed shifted.[14]

CUSP has evolved. In contrast to the original 8 steps, the current CUSP framework involves prework activities followed by 5 core steps.[11] The process, which is intended to be ongoing and cyclical, also incorporates timely data feedback and periodic check-ins with the team to identify challenges and needs.[11] **Fig. 1** depicts the contemporary CUSP framework.

The first broad implementation of CUSP began in 2003 as the Keystone ICU Project.[16] More than 100 ICUs, most of which were located in Michigan, participated in an interventional study aimed at reducing catheter-related BSIs.[16] These ICUs implemented 5 interventions directly aimed at reducing targeted infections, along with CUSP to improve the culture of safety, and tools to improve clinician-to-clinician communication.[17] Outcomes included a reduction from mean baseline infection rates of 7.7 per 1000 catheter days to follow-up rates of 1.4 infections per 1000 catheter days at 16 to 18 months.[17]

Another measure of the Keystone ICU Project was assessment of teamwork climate, for which 72 ICUs submitted pre-CUSP and post-CUSP data.[18] Analysis found a statistically significant improvement in teamwork climate for the sample, with a shift from 17% reporting positive teamwork at baseline to 46% the following year; however, not all units improved. Not surprisingly, conflict resolution, nurse input and nurse-physician input were rated much lower in units with lower post-CUSP teamwork climate scores but trended positively with ICUs improving scores by10 or more points.[18]

To add strength to the Keystone Project findings, another study using a robust, multicenter, phased, cluster-randomized controlled design occurred in 45 ICUs across 35 different hospitals around the United States.[19] This study of a nurse-led program, completed in 2008, found the combination of evidence-based practices (EBP) and CUSP had a causal relationship with fewer central line-associated BSIs in both

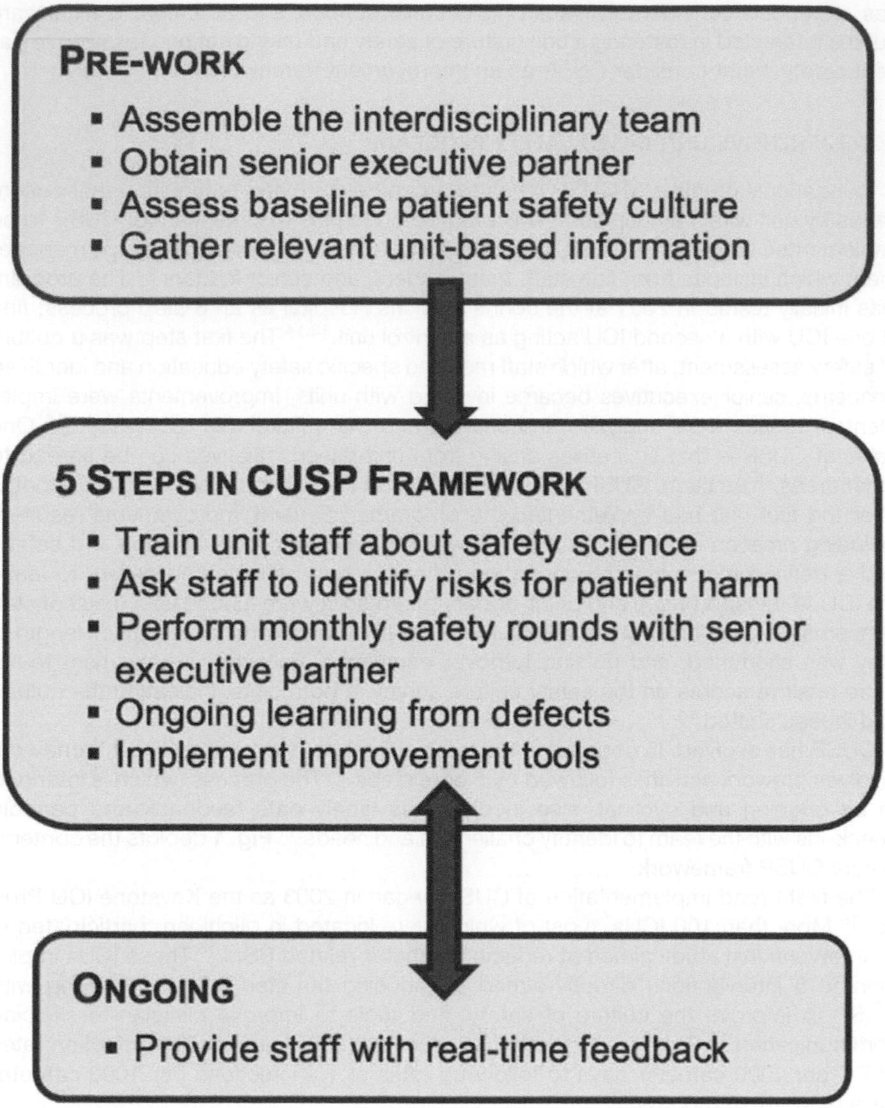

PRE-WORK

- Assemble the interdisciplinary team
- Obtain senior executive partner
- Assess baseline patient safety culture
- Gather relevant unit-based information

5 STEPS IN CUSP FRAMEWORK

- Train unit staff about safety science
- Ask staff to identify risks for patient harm
- Perform monthly safety rounds with senior executive partner
- Ongoing learning from defects
- Implement improvement tools

ONGOING

- Provide staff with real-time feedback

Fig. 1. Outline of steps before, during, and after CUSP kickoff. (*Adapted from* Johns Hopkins Medicine Center for Innovation in Quality Patient Care. Five steps of CUSP. Available at: http://www.hopkinsmedicine.org/innovation_quality_patient_care/areas_expertise/improve_patient_safety/cusp/five_steps_cusp.html. Accessed November 7, 2013. Used with permission.)

the intervention (81% reduction) and control (69% reduction) groups. The researchers noted the value nurse leadership brought to this quality improvement project's success.[19]

Since the Keystone project, similar work has spread in the effort to eliminate BSIs. AHRQ and private philanthropists funded a national program called, "On the CUSP: Stop BSI," which used CUSP and other tactics described in the Keystone project, along with a model of translating research into practice.[20] Several states implemented the program. For example, on the CUSP: Stop BSI implementation began in Hawaii in 2009.[21] All acute care hospitals in Hawaii that had adult ICU beds participated, implementing CUSP and specific interventions for central line care. The mean rate of central line–associated BSIs decreased by 61%, from 1.5 infections per 1000 catheter days to 0.6 infections per 1000 catheter days, 16 to 18 months after project implementation. The researchers emphasized the importance of CUSP in creating a culture of safety to promote adoption of quality improvement activities.[21] The Hawaiian initiative later spread to clinical units beyond adult ICUs, including medical/surgical units, operating rooms, emergency departments, and pediatric and neonatal ICUs.[22] The program was implemented in other states as well. In Connecticut, 17 participating ICUs were able to achieve a 41% decline in central line BSI.[23] Although the results did not reach statistical significance, BSI reduction was viewed positively and further supported the use of CUSP coupled with other interventions.[23]

BSIs are not the only issue tackled by CUSP teams, and improvements have been implemented in several types of clinical units. For instance, a nurse manager and surgeon led a team to implement CUSP on a surgical unit with support from a CUSP coach and a senior executive.[24] Interdisciplinary unit team members, including licensed and unlicensed staff, were invited to monthly CUSP meetings. Safety concerns were identified and prioritized, and then tools to improve communication, team collaboration, and safer care were put into practice. Authors described CUSP as a platform to empower staff to solve safety problems. Postimplementation survey results compared with those collected pre-CUSP reflected more positive perceptions of teamwork (10% increase) and safety (23% increase). Nurse turnover decreased over the same timeframe.[24]

Elsewhere, in obstetrics, CUSP has been used as a vehicle to drive improvements in patient safety culture and perinatal care processes.[25] Although the obstetric project was successful in achieving desired improvements, the investigators reported challenges in getting buy-in from some clinicians and concluded that ongoing encouragement and administrative support are helpful in creating change.

In a different population and setting, an interdisciplinary team caring for colorectal surgery patients in Maryland implemented CUSP and select interventions to reduce surgical site infections.[26] After this CUSP project, the mean rate of surgical site infections decreased by 33.3%. The authors acknowledged the value of local wisdom of front-line providers on the team to make improvements in patient safety.[26]

AHRQ has embraced CUSP and awarded more than $8,000,000 to expand and implement CUSP projects nationally.[27] In addition to BSI reduction, funded CUSP projects focus on catheter-associated urinary tract infection prevention, evaluation of practices around different types of catheter locks in dialysis patients, and prevention of ventilator-associated pneumonia.[27,28] Progress reports about AHRQ CUSP initiatives may be found on the agency's Web site at: www.ahrq.gov/professionals/quality-patient-safety/cusp/index.html.

Resources are available to guide those interested in exploring CUSP further. CUSP information and tools can be found by accessing the Web sites listed in **Box 1**. Additionally, Pronovost and colleagues[12] described how a Web-based tool can be used to support organizations' use of CUSP. In one example, the Web-based tool was used by a team to improve patient arm-banding processes at a medical birthing center so patients could be positively identified.[12] This tool also was used by a medical progressive care unit team to ensure intravenous tubing changes occurred appropriately, along with a project aiming to improve physician-nurse communication.[12]

Aforementioned projects show the flexibility to use CUSP in different clinical settings to address an array of safety improvement opportunities. Benefits impact

---

Box 1
Web sites with CUSP information

The Agency for Healthcare Research and Quality

- http://www.ahrq.gov/professionals/education/curriculum-tools/cusptoolkit/modules/learn/index.html

Johns Hopkins Medicine Center for Innovation in Quality Patient Care

- http://www.hopkinsmedicine.org/innovation_quality_patient_care/areas_expertise/improve_patient_safety/cusp/

---

patients directly and foster teamwork and empower bedside staff to speak up and lead change. Organizational benefits include reductions in adverse events and lower nurse turnover.

ONE INTENSIVE CARE UNIT'S EXPERIENCE WITH COMPREHENSIVE UNIT-BASED SAFETY PROGRAM

The first CUSP in the authors' hospital premiered in the cardiovascular ICU (CVICU) in 2010 with support from the health care system, hospital, and unit-level leaders. The hospital is a large, urban, tertiary-care, academic medical center located in the south-central United States. The 24-bed CVICU serves a primary population of cardio-thoracic surgery, ventricular-assist device implantation, heart transplant, and lung transplant patients. The hospital's chief nursing officer engaged as the unit's senior executive partner. CUSP prework done by unit leaders including the nurse manager, supervisors, and educator involved collecting a baseline culture assessment and inviting interdisciplinary team members to participate in CUSP. Staff received education about CUSP, and then the team began meeting every 2 weeks to identify opportunities to improve patient safety.

COMPREHENSIVE UNIT-BASED SAFETY PROGRAM: SPARKING THE INTEREST FOR PATIENT SAFETY

Because of the grassroots nature of CUSP, nurses were encouraged to have open dialogue with the interdisciplinary team regarding safety concerns and to recommend solutions. Significant dissatisfaction with the postoperative handover process between the anesthesia provider and the ICU nurse surfaced as an area of concern. Team members proposed making changes to the existing handover process. They thought an improvement in communications would reduce risks of medication and other types of errors and also contribute to a healthy work environment. Additionally, the nurses believed by strengthening the handover process between the anesthesia provider and the receiving nurse, the plan of care would be clearer, and the nurse would be better equipped to address individual patient needs.

The nurses' perception that the handover process of postoperative patients has significant safety implications is well supported by literature categorizing the handover as a critical time of transferring information and responsibility. Handover failures are a large source of medical error; therefore, opportunities for improvement must be identified and rectified.[29] Cardiac surgery patients may be particularly vulnerable because of the risk of hemodynamic instability during the transition from the operating room (OR) to the ICU.[30] These patients are highly complex and defenseless, as they are most often sedated, thus, communication errors may have serious and potentially grave consequences.[30,31]

Other factors can also impact safety of handovers, such as the consistency of what is contained in the information exchange. Issues including turnover of health care team members and shift work are risks inherent to the health care setting.[29,32] Ensuring high-quality information is consistently provided during handoffs not only helps mitigate threats to safety but also minimizes rework by nurses left with inaccurate or inadequate patient information.[29]

Unfortunately, gaps in communication continue to have serious consequences. The Joint Commission collects and periodically publishes data on root causes of significant errors. For the first half of calendar year 2013, the top 2 root causes of errors included human factors, such as fatigue and distraction, and communication failures.[33] Both of these factors can pose risks during the postoperative handover. A typical verbal handover includes complex, detailed information about the patient's history, operative course, and current status. Distractions can occur during this transfer of care, partially because of the beehivelike atmosphere at the bedside on the patient's initial arrival into the ICU. Multiple team members typically converge to assist with patient care activities and settle the patient into the unit, attending to tasks such as connecting monitoring devices, administering intravenous medications and fluids, adjusting ventilator settings, drawing blood, and entering data into the electronic health record. Given these circumstances, it was no surprise that breakdowns in communication during handoffs were a patient safety concern of the CVICU team.

During a review of relevant literature, several sources were found to support use of a standardized handover tool. The main purpose for all patient handovers is to accurately transfer information about each patient's situation and care plan, thereby ensuring patient safety and continuity of care.[29] Experts have promoted the value of standardized handover processes in high-stakes situations. Some lessons have come from other industries in which teams effectively use standardized processes to promote safety. For example, the aviation and motor racing industries have been leaders in exemplifying how teams can effectively work together in complex situations with minimal time or room for error. Drawing on the safety expertise of aviation and racing professionals, a team in the United Kingdom developed and implemented a postsurgery handover protocol.[34] After implementing the protocol, errors decreased significantly and teamwork improved. The authors expressed a unique need in health care for an easily understood and trainable handover process secondary to high turnover of health care workers.[34] Another investigation of a structured handover protocol yielded similar results. The protocol, used when pediatric cardiac surgery patients are moved from the OR to the ICU, resulted in improved teamwork, significantly fewer technical errors, and a reduction in omission of critical information without adding time.[30] More recently, a report showed how use of a single page tool outlining information to be exchanged during postoperative handover of pediatric cardiac surgery patients improved the quality of information exchanged without requiring more time.[31] There was also a trend toward fewer high-risk events after the handover process was implemented.[31] A clear, transparent, and comprehensive handover process minimizes the likelihood of error.[29]

ACTING ON OPPORTUNITIES FOR IMPROVEMENT

The CVICU CUSP team was aware of the pitfalls associated with handovers and desired practical solutions. Once the need for change was identified, everyone was eager to share suggestions to correct potential safety issues. The interdisciplinary team set to work identifying specific opportunities related to the handover from the OR to the ICU. Team members included several staff nurses, the unit's nurse manager, a unit supervisor, an anesthesiologist, a respiratory care practitioner, and unit-based pharmacists, with the chief nursing officer as the executive partner. The culture promoted by the CUSP philosophy allowed team members to stay focused on the central purpose of enhancing patient safety during postoperative transfer of care from one caregiver to another. The hospital's nursing professional practice model, which emphasizes the nurse's role in creating safe passage for patients, also guided the team's intentions.[35]

One of the authors, then a staff nurse, became the project leader and shared information gleaned from the review of literature with the team. The team supported the concept of a standardized handover process. Nurses and anesthesia providers identified optimal elements for an ideal postoperative handover, which are summarized in **Box 2**. Key themes involved intravenous medication safety, communication expectations, and being adequately prepared to care for the patient. The primary goal was to standardize the handover process to ensure each patient was consistently and safely received into the ICU. The team decided to create a communication tool in the form of a checklist to aid in establishing well-defined roles and expectations for all participants in the handover and to clearly convey the plan of care for the patient. The new methodology of handover was dubbed the *Royal Exchange*.

Now that there was an action plan, the team needed to determine what to include on the checklist. A report of experiences from a successful pilot of a postoperative handover protocol from the OR to ICU emphasized the importance of relaying a patient's most significant risk of harm during the process.[36] Based on this, discussions were held among staff nurses, other nursing leaders, pharmacists, a system patient safety consultant and human factors specialist, and anesthesiologists to determine which aspects of the handover process were most likely to result in error or compromise safety. Team members' comments were compiled and compared with best practices found in the literature. The team reached consensus on specific issues they proposed become part of the postoperative handover process. They developed the Royal Exchange checklist, outlining significant pieces of information essential for a patient's safe passage (**Fig. 2**). In addition, a teaching tool was created by the project leader to inform staff how to use the checklist.

PROCESS IMPLEMENTATION

The ICU nurses responsible for admitting cardiac surgery patients received education to prepare for the process change. Education included face-to-face interactions with

---

Box 2
CUSP team's list: optimal elements of an ideal handover

- ICU room setup will be consistent and contain equipment for extubation and oxygenation
- Intravenous pumps and tubing will be labeled for safe administration of medicated drips
- Primary RN will introduce self as such to anesthesia
- Monitoring devices will be connected in order consistent with best practice
- Report will be standardized and include patient's baseline status, any complications of case, and plan of care
- Core measures will be discussed
- Nurse will be afforded an opportunity to clarify report and plan of care
- Anesthesia provider will provide contact information in case questions or needs arise

Date: _____

ICU RN: _____

Anesthesia: _____

Contact Info: _____

Nursing

	Prior to Admission:
	Room and **hallway** clear
	Family in waiting area
	Ventilator set-up in room
	Suction canister with **Yankauer**
	Ambu bag, Nasal cannula, Venti-mask

	Admission:
	Primary RN introduces self
	Monitoring connected in correct order:
	1. Pulse oximetry
	2. Arterial line BP
	3. ECG
	4. NIBP (only if requested or no a-line)
	5. Core temp
	Vitals verbalized and agreed upon
	Drip and safety check
	Wait to change IVF or clean lines
	Seek clarification if needed before anesthesia leaves

Place patient label here:

Anesthesia

	Prior to ICU Admission:
	Pumps programmed appropriately
	Pumps labeled
	Standard or MAX concentration of drips used
	Sedation drips with patient if to be continued
	Claves and caps on exposed inlets

	Report:
	Operation performed--Please be specific.
	Do we suspect any complications?
	Brief patient history
	Height & Weight
	Allergies
	Co-morbidities and previous surgeries
	Systems Report
	CV: ischemia, arrhythmias
	Blood Products: given and availability
	Pulmonary
	Neuro: abnormal base line, psych hx, addictions
	Renal
	GI: bariatric sx, contraindications to NGT
	Labs (Hct, K, baseline Cr, coagulopathies, ABG)
	Plan
	Extubation plan
	Bleeding issues
	Blood pressure (stability, goal BP?)
	Drugs (weaning, IVPs given affecting sedation/BP, etc.)
	Pain control
	Core Measures
	Glucose
	Antibiotic Start Time
	ASA for AMI

	Recommendations
	Ask for questions and comfort level of RN
	Anesthesia provider contact information

THIS DOCUMENT IS NOT PART OF THE PERMANENT RECORD

Version 1.3

Fig. 2. The Royal Exchange checklist. (*Used with permission from* Baylor University Medical Center, Dallas, TX.)

the team leader along with documents describing the Royal Exchange and how to use the checklist. To complement the nurse education, an anesthesiologist educated the anesthesia providers.

The robust process has now been in place in the CVICU for almost 3 years. A staff nurse's perspective of the current postoperative handover is presented in **Box 3**. The ICU nurses are responsible for initiating the checklist before receipt of the patient by completing the section detailing room set-up expectations. At the time of patient admission, the nurse completes the remainder of the checklist as each expected handover component is fulfilled. Completed checklists are stored in a binder on the unit and reviewed periodically to validate the expected handover process has been completed with each admission. In congruence with the idea of CUSP as an ongoing process, the Royal Exchange checklist has been refined over time.

> **Box 3**
> **An RN's perspective of the handover process using the Royal Exchange**
>
> ## The handoff experience from the view of the bedside RN
>
> Kelsey, RN prepares room with the designated supplies and ensures all necessary equipment for extubation is at the bedside. She makes sure the halls are clear and the pathway from the OR is free from objects.
>
> As the patient rolls in, the Royal Exchange begins. Kelsey assesses the stability of the patient who just had a coronary artery bypass of vessels and a mitral valve replacement. She connects the patient to the monitor in the appropriate order. The recorder in the room verifies with the anesthesia provider synchronicity of the vital signs, which are then entered into the electronic health record.
>
> After adjusting any drips to maintain hemodynamic stability, Kelsey performs a drip and safety check. Nurses now expect anesthesia to label the IV lines and pumps and program the drips into the pump library using only the standard or maximum drip concentrations. The drip check is much simpler now and promotes a very safe environment for the nurse to administer intravenous medications.
>
> Now begins the report. The anesthesia provider starts by stating the operation and any specific complications that may have occurred or that Kelsey may need to anticipate. He discusses the patient in a systematic manner that is easily followed. He then goes into the plan for the patient regarding extubation, bleeding, weaning medicated drips, vital sign parameters, and pain control. The anesthesia provider also discusses core measures, such as aspirin administration, if the patient was admitted with an acute myocardial infarction, blood glucose control, and antibiotic start time.
>
> Before the anesthesia provider leaves, Kelsey is afforded an opportunity to ask questions and clarify the plan of care. Anesthesia also provides contact information should she think of a question later.
>
> Kelsey is satisfied that she is able to safely care for her patient. The patient remains sedated, vulnerable, and unaware of the exchange of information, but he has been safely transferred from the operating room to the intensive care unit as a result of the Royal Exchange.

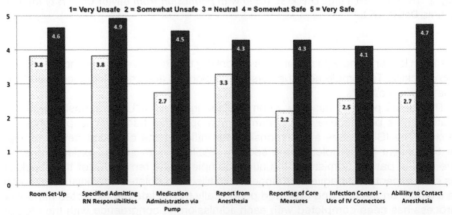

Fig. 3. Pre- and postsurvey results for safety of the patient.

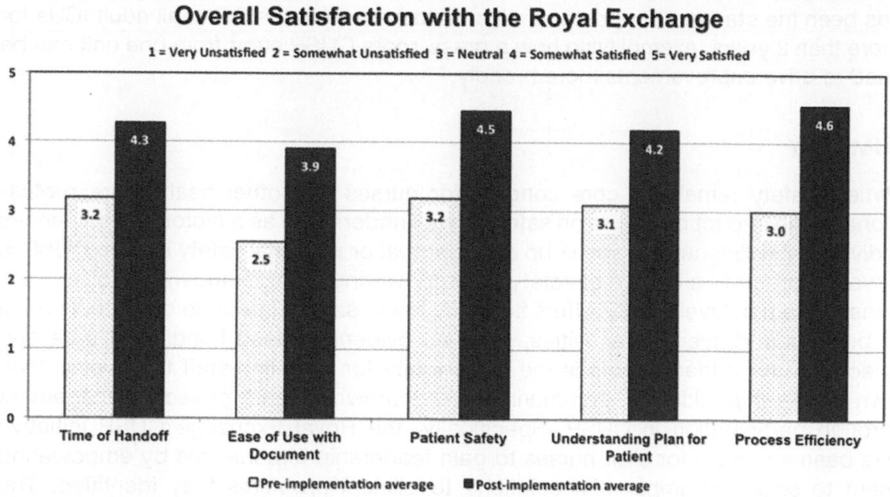

Overall Satisfaction with the Royal Exchange

1 = Very Unsatisfied 2 = Somewhat Unsatisfied 3 = Neutral 4 = Somewhat Satisfied 5= Very Satisfied

Category	Pre-implementation average	Post-implementation average
Time of Handoff	3.2	4.3
Ease of Use with Document	2.5	3.9
Patient Safety	3.2	4.5
Understanding Plan for Patient	3.1	4.2
Process Efficiency	3.0	4.6

☐ Pre-implementation average   ■ Post-implementation average

Fig. 4. Pre- and postsurvey results for overall satisfaction.

OUTCOMES

Pre- and postimplementation data were collected to assess the nurses' perceptions of patient safety around 7 specific handover issues. Results (**Fig. 3**) show an improved mean rating for all issues. Nurses also rated their overall satisfaction with the handover process before and after implementation of the Royal Exchange (**Fig. 4**), and findings reflect increased satisfaction for all items measured. The anesthesiologists also expressed high satisfaction with the initiative. Benefits of the Royal Exchange to nurses, anesthesiologists, and patients are outlined in **Box 4**. Through the leadership of front-line nurses and other health care professionals engaged in CUSP, the unit's culture shifted, and a new safety practice became a common expectation of all members of the team.

Because of these successes, it was proposed the Royal Exchange spread to the other 6 adult ICUs in the hospital to standardize this best practice. The checklist

---

Box 4
Benefits of the Royal Exchange to designated stakeholders

Nurse	• Clear plan of care for the patient
	• Consistent report
	• Intravenous medications easily recognized and safely administered
	• Information needed to contact anesthesia if any questions arise after admission
Anesthesiologist	• Room set-up consistent
	• Primary nurse easily identified
	• Order of monitor connections consistent with best practice
Patient	• Patient safely transferred from care of the anesthesia provider into the intensive care unit
	• All relevant information including core measures discussed and the nurse has the information necessary to provide safe care

has been the standard for postoperative handovers from the OR to all adult ICUs for more than 2 years, exemplifying how a grass-roots CUSP effort from one unit can be used to drive improvements more broadly.

SUMMARY

Patient safety remains a core concern for nurses and other health care professionals. The impact of culture on safety is well understood as a factor that influences individuals' willingness to speak up about actual or potential safety issues. CUSP is a way to promote a culture of safety by empowering team members to solve problems at the unit level. CUSP offers flexibility necessary to integrate other tools used in process improvement activities, such as evidence-based bundles of care and checklists. An added benefit is the opportunity for front-line staff to develop their own leadership skills in communication, teamwork, and project management through participation in CUSP. Specifically, the Royal Exchange CUSP initiative has been a vehicle for staff nurses to gain leadership experiences by empowering them to seek and implement solutions to clinical problems they identified. The CUSP approach links beautifully with the concept of nursing as a complex adaptive system, in which formal leaders need to foster leadership in everyone.[3] With this mindset, nurses at all levels can respond innovatively and independently to challenges that arise.[3] Although gaps in health care quality and safety remain, nurses who choose to engage in activities aimed at closing those gaps, such as CUSP, undoubtedly will be instrumental in creating meaningful changes for the benefit of patients and health care professionals alike.

REFERENCES

1. Kohn LT, Corrigan JM, Donaldson SS, editors. To err is human: building a safer health system. Washington, DC: National Academies Press; 1999.
2. Wachter RM. Patient safety at ten: unmistakable progress, troubling gaps. Health Aff 2010;29(1):165–73. http://dx.doi.org/10.1377/hlthaff.2009.0785.
3. Chafee MW, McNeill MM. A model of nursing as a complex adaptive system. Nurs Outlook 2007;55(5):232–41. http://dx.doi.org/10.1016/j.outlook.2007.04.003. Available at: http://c.ymcdn.com/sites/www.plexusinstitute.org/resource/collection/24E190C9-B485-4256-BDD5-10548A9FF0C4/Chaffee_-_Nursing_As_CAS_-_Nursing_Outlook_2007.pdf.
4. Chassin MR. Improving the quality of health care: what's taking so long? Health Aff 2013;32(10):1761–5. http://dx.doi.org/10.1377/hlthaff.2013.0809.
5. Resar R, Griffin FA, Haraden C, et al. Using care bundles to improve health care quality. IHI innovation series white paper. Cambridge (MA): Institute for Healthcare Improvement; 2012. Available at: http://www.ihi.org/knowledge/Pages/IHIWhitePapers/UsingCareBundles.aspx. Accessed November 6, 2013.
6. Implement the IHI Ventilator Bundle. Institute for Healthcare Improvement Web site. 2011. Available at: http://www.ihi.org/knowledge/Pages/Changes/ImplementtheVentilatorBundle.aspx. Accessed November 6, 2013.
7. Patient Safety Checklists. The World Health Organization Web site. Available at: http://www.who.int/patientsafety/implementation/checklists/en/. Accessed November 7, 2013.
8. Chassin MR, Loeb JM. High reliability health care: getting there from here. Milbank Q 2013;91(3):459–90. Available at: http://onlinelibrary.wiley.com/doi/10.1111/1468-0009.12023/pdf.

9. TeamSTEPPS: National Implementation. Agency for Healthcare Research and Quality Web site. Available at: http://teamstepps.ahrq.gov/about-2cl_3.htm. Accessed November 6, 2013.

10. Fact sheet: ending healthcare-associated infections. Agency for Healthcare Research and Quality Web site. 2009. Available at: http://www.ahrq.gov/research/findings/factsheets/errors-safety/haicusp/haicusp.pdf. Accessed November 6, 2013.

11. The Comprehensive Unit-based Safety Program. Johns Hopkins Medicine Web site. Available at: http://www.hopkinsmedicine.org/innovation_quality_patient_care/areas_expertise/improve_patient_safety/cusp/. Accessed November 7, 2013.

12. Pronovost PJ, King J, Holzmueller CG, et al. A web-based tool for the comprehensive unit-based safety program (CUSP). Jt Comm J Qual Patient Saf 2006;32(3):119–29.

13. Pronovost PJ, Berenholtz SM, Goeschel CA, et al. Creating high reliability in health care organizations. Health Serv Res 2006;41(4 Pt 2):1599–617. http://dx.doi.org/10.1111/j.1475-6773.2006.00567.x.

14. Pronovost P, Weast B, Rosenstein B, et al. Implementing and validating a comprehensive unit-based safety program. J Patient Saf 2005;1(1):33–40.

15. Pronovost P, Holzmueller CG. Partnering for quality. J Crit Care 2004;19(3):121–9. http://dx.doi.org/10.1016/j.jcrc.2004.07.004.

16. Using a comprehensive unit-based safety program to prevent healthcare-associated infections. Agency for Healthcare Research and Quality Web site. 2013. Available at: http://www.ahrq.gov/professionals/quality-patient-safety/cusp/index.html. Accessed November 7, 2013.

17. Pronovost P, Needham D, Berenholtz S, et al. An intervention to decrease catheter-related bloodstream infections in the ICU. N Engl J Med 2006;355(26):2725–32. http://dx.doi.org/10.1056/NEJMoa061115.

18. Pronovost PJ, Berenholtz SM, Goeschel C, et al. Improving patient safety in intensive care units in Michigan. J Crit Care 2008;23(2):207–21. http://dx.doi.org/10.1016/j.jcrc.2007.09.002.

19. Marstellar JA, Sexton JB, Hsu YJ, et al. A multicenter, phased, cluster-randomized controlled trial to reduce central line-associated bloodstream infections in intensive care units. Crit Care Med 2012;40(100):2933–9. http://dx.doi.org/10.1097/CCM.0b013e31825fd4d8.

20. Sawyer M, Weeks C, Goeschel CA, et al. Using evidence, rigorous measurement, and collaboration to eliminate central catheter-associated bloodstream infections. Crit Care Med 2010;38(Suppl 8):S292–8. http://dx.doi.org/10.1097/CCM.0b013e3181e6a165.

21. Lin DM, Weeks K, Bauer L, et al. Eradicating central line-associated bloodstream infections statewide: the Hawaii experience. Am J Med Qual 2012;27(2):124–9. http://dx.doi.org/10.1177/1062860611414299.

22. Lin DM, Weeks K, Holzmueller CG, et al. Maintaining and sustaining the on the CUSP: stop BSI model in Hawaii. Jt Comm J Qual Patient Saf 2013;39(2):51–60.

23. Hong AL, Sawyer MD, Shore A, et al. Decreasing central-line-associated bloodstream infections in Connecticut intensive care units. J Healthc Qual 2013;35(5):78–87. http://dx.doi.org/10.1111/j.1945-1474.2012.00210.x.

24. Timmel J, Kent P, Holzmueller CG, et al. Impact of the comprehensive unit-based safety program (CUSP) on safety culture in a surgical inpatient unit. Jt Comm J Qual Patient Saf 2010;36(6):252–60.

25. Simpson KR, Knox GE, Martin M, et al. Michigan Health & Hospital Association Keystone Obstetrics: a statewide collaborative for perinatal patient safety in Michigan. Jt Comm J Qual Patient Saf 2011;37(12):544–52.
26. Wick EC, Hobson DB, Bennett JL, et al. Implementation of a surgical comprehensive unit-based safety program to reduce surgical site infections. J Am Coll Surg 2012;215(2):193–200. http://dx.doi.org/10.1016/j.jamcollsurg.2012.03.017.
27. Ending Health Care-Associated Infections. Agency for Healthcare Research and Quality Web site. 2010. Available at: http://www.ahrq.gov/research/findings/factsheets/errors-safety/haicusp/index.html#projcusp. Accessed November 7, 2013.
28. AHRQ Project to Prevent Healthcare-Associated Infection, Fiscal Year 2011. Agency for Healthcare Research and Quality Web site. 2010. Available at: http://www.ahrq.gov/research/findings/factsheets/errors-safety/haify11/index.html. Accessed November 7, 2013.
29. Nagpal K, Arora S, Abboudi M, et al. Postoperative handover: problems, pitfalls, and prevention of error. Ann Surg 2010;252(1):171–6. http://dx.doi.org/10.1097/SLA.0b013e3181dc3656.
30. Joy BF, Elliott E, Hardy C, et al. Standardized multidisciplinary protocol improves handover of cardiac surgery patients to the intensive care unit. Pediatr Crit Care Med 2011;12(3):304–8. http://dx.doi.org/10.1097/PCC.0b013e3181fe25a1.
31. Zavalkoff S, Razack S, Lavoie J, et al. Handover after pediatric heart surgery: a simple tool improves information exchange. Pediatr Crit Care Med 2011;12: 309–13. http://dx.doi.org/10.1097/PCC.0b013e3181fe27b6.
32. Halm M. Nursing handoffs: ensuring safe passage for patients. Am J Crit Care 2013;22:158–62. http://dx.doi.org/10.4037/ajcc2013454.
33. The Joint Commission. Sentinel event statistics for First Half of 2013. Joint Commission Perspective 2013;33(10):1–3. Available at: http://mail.tcrespite.com/TJCNewsletters/Perspectives/Perspectives-10.pdf.
34. Catchpole K, de Leval M, McEwan A, et al. Patient handover from surgery to intensive care: using formula 1 pit-stop and aviation models to improve safety and quality. Paediatr Anaesth 2007;17:470–8. http://dx.doi.org/10.1111/j.1460-9592.2007.02239.x.
35. Bradley DA, Dixon J. Staff nurses creating safe passage with evidence-based practice. Nurs Clin North Am 2009;44(1):71–81. http://dx.doi.org/10.1016/j.cnur.2008.10.002.
36. Petrovic M, Aboumatar H, Baumgartner W, et al. Pilot implementation of a perioperative protocol to guide operating room-to-intensive care unit patient handoffs. J Cardiothorac Vasc Anesth 2012;26(1):11–6. http://dx.doi.org/10.1053/j.jvca.2011.07.009.

Incidence and Prevention of Delirium in Critical Care Patients

Megan Wheeler, MSN, RN, ACNS-BC[a],*,
Carol Crenshaw, MBA, BSN, RN[b],
Sharon Gunn, MSN, MA, RN, ACNS-BC, CCRN[a]

KEYWORDS

- Delirium • Intensive care • Complex adaptive system • Delirium screening

KEY POINTS

- Delirium in the intensive care unit is a very prevalent issue.
- Process improvement projects can be performed successfully around prevention of and screening for delirium.
- Even with these projects, awareness, and educational materials, delirium remains hard to treat.

INTRODUCTION

As much as nurses would love to think of their delirious patients in regards to Merriam-Webster's secondary definition, "a state of wild excitement and great happiness,"[1] it is not the case with critical care patients. These patients have a wide variety of causes of their delirium, treatment plans, and long-term outcomes. Delirium has been studied and written about a great deal, and the disease process may very well be a complex adaptive system in itself. This article discusses delirium screening and prevention at a major health system.

REVIEW OF LITERATURE

Literature searches were performed in both Medline and CINAHL databases. It seems as if a plethora of literature exists on delirium, particularly delirium in Critical Care. References from previous evidence-based practice projects within this health care system related to delirium were also examined.

The authors have nothing to disclose.
[a] Baylor Health Care System at Dallas, 2001 Bryan Street, Ste 600, Dallas, TX 75201, USA;
[b] Baylor University Medical Center at Dallas, 3500 Gaston Avenue, Dallas, TX 75246, USA
* Corresponding author.
E-mail address: megan.wheeler@baylorhealth.edu

Crit Care Nurs Clin N Am 26 (2014) 461–468
http://dx.doi.org/10.1016/j.ccell.2014.08.003
0899-5885/14/$ – see front matter © 2014 Elsevier Inc. All rights reserved.

The key feature used to define delirium is inattention that happens suddenly and oscillates over time.[2] "It is the inattention that appears to be the hallmark and pivotal feature of delirium."[2] It is accompanied by either disorganized thinking or a change in level of consciousness, or both. There are 3 subtypes of delirium: hypoactive, hyperactive, and a combination of both.[3] It has been determined that the acute illness process probably precipitates hypoactive delirium,[1,4–6] while effects on neurotransmitters provided by drugs, chemicals, and anticholinergic agents are more likely to cause hyperactive delirium.[1,7–9]

There are multiple risk factors for delirium and these risks can mostly be grouped into precipitating factors and predisposing factors. It is said that the relationship between these factors is what determines the likelihood of onset of delirium.[1] Some of these risk factors include older age, established cognitive impairment, numerous acute illnesses, and numerous medications.[10] Delirium also has significant long-term effects, "including increased mortality, persistent cognitive impairment with functional decline, and an increase in nursing home placements after discharge."[11–15] Another study revealed that delirium can increase the risk of developing dementia.[16]

Delirium in the intensive care unit (ICU) is associated with numerous negative outcomes, attributing to higher health care costs. Literature has revealed that delirium can be linked with a 31% increase in overall hospital costs and a 39% increase in ICU costs.[15,17] In 2008, it was estimated that annual costs in the United States could reach $152 billion.[15,18] In a study that recruited patients and then looked at their records in the 4 years before the index admission and followed their records for 5 years after the index admission, it was noted that patients with delirium had an elevated risk of death and hospital admission for up to 5 years after the initial episode.[19]

Researchers agree that prevention is crucial in decreasing delirium. Multiple studies focused on prevention of delirium concentrate on educating staff, consulting experts, and protocols that seek out multiple risk factors.[15,20–22] This major health system focused on the same type of interventions for delirium prevention.

CASE STUDY 1

A process improvement project was taken on at the authors' facility to increase awareness and delirium screening by ICU nursing staff. This case study reviews the process improvement project.

In reviewing the literature, it was noted that up to 90% of ICU patients were found to be positive for delirium. Delirium increases morbidity, mortality, costs, and length of stay for critically ill patients. Delirium has long-term ramifications on the patient's functional and mental status. At a university medical center, it was identified that patients in the ICU were not being screened with a standardized tool.

A multidisciplinary team was formed for a process improvement project with the goals of

1. Implementing delirium screening using the confusion assessment method intensive care unit (CAM-ICU) screening tool
2. Implementing an order set to help prevent and treat patients with delirium

A medical intensive care unit (MICU) was selected as the pilot unit to reduce the incidence of delirium. In the first Plan Do Check Act cycle, selected registered nurses were trained as supertrainers to do the initial baseline delirium screening using the CAM-ICU tool. There are essentially 2 steps to be taken when performing the CAM-ICU. During the first step, the patient's sedation level is assessed. Patients who are deeply sedated, not arousable, combative, or agitated are excluded from the second step. In the second step, the patient is asked to perform a series of tasks. The patient is scored on the ability to successfully complete these tasks. Ability to perform the tasks allows the nurse to reliably determine whether the patient has delirium.

Nurses specially educated on how to perform delirium screenings using the CAM-ICU conducted the screenings using the tool and collected data on predisposing and precipitating factors for delirium for each patient on a tracking sheet that was developed to record their results. The data obtained were analyzed to determine the baseline rate of delirium. In the second cycle of the project, in-services were organized for all staff nurses about incidence, causes, and patient outcomes related to delirium. Education was also provided on why a valid and reliable screening tool was necessary for screening. Staff was taught the importance of accurate, consistent screening, and how to use the CAM-ICU screening tool. After training, all staff nurses conducted the screening with their patient assessments and documented the results on the Vital Sign Flow Sheet. Two supertrainers were available on all nursing shifts as resources for any questions that arose. Supertrainers, ICU supervisors, and the clinical nurse specialist randomly screened patients with staff nurses to insure accuracy of screening. Charge nurses tallied the results from the Vital Sign Flow Sheet to the Delirium Tracking Sheet to track the number of patients positive, negative, and unable to screen according to the CAM-ICU. From that information, the incidence of delirium was determined.

In the third cycle of the project, additional education for staff nurses was conducted to hardwire the CAM-ICU screening process and implement the evidenced-based order set (Fig. 1). The order set was developed by an interprofessional group consisting of staff nurse input and collaboration with the clinical nurse specialist, pharmacist, and ICU intensivist. The order set was vetted through several multidisciplinary groups before being finalized and implemented.

Unit staff was informed of the new order set and the evidence-based practices it contained. Initially, the incidence of delirium and use of the order set were discussed during intensivist-led multidisciplinary rounds on a daily basis. Ongoing education was provided for all staff nurses on an "as-needed" basis to provide consistency in the CAM-ICU screening tool and use of the order set.

METRICS

Once initial data were obtained, implementation of evidence-based interventions occurred from October 2010 to February 2011. Screenings of patients before the implementation demonstrated that 42% of all of the MICU patients were positive for delirium when screened with the CAM-ICU tool by staff trained how to use the tool. The goal was further expanded to include a decrease in the number of patients with delirium by 10% of the baseline positive screenings obtained. To achieve this goal, no more than 37.8% of patients would have delirium after implementation of the interventions.

The outcome of the process improvement project showed a decrease in the percentage of patients with delirium in this MICU from 42% when the delirium order set was introduced to 23% during the time frame of this project (November 15 through December 31, 2010). The lessons learned included the following:

- Delirium screening process needs to be hardwired to ensure accurate data
- Physician education is needed to promote use of the order set
- Electronic Health Record documentation is needed to support staff compliance
- "Buy in" from all involved employees from the beginning stages helps with the results. Continuous feedback and reinforcement are necessary.

- Collaboration with IT is being done so that the Electronic Health Record can support the document and run reports. Long-term outcomes related to length of stay, ventilator days, and mortality are to be tracked.

The project led to several outcomes that had system-wide implications: delirium screening and practices to reduce the incidence of delirium (or minimize delirium days) were spread throughout the health care system's critical care units. Several staff nurses from the Medical ICU created a video with the clinical nurse specialist entitled, "What Is Delirium." One staff nurse completed a project on delirium. A trial pilot on one of the facility's medicine floors was a spinoff of this project. Several national presentations resulted from the project.

PHYSICIAN ORDERS

Delirium ICU Order Set

Activity
- ☐ Bedrest with passive range of motion
- ☐ Bedrest with bedside commode
- ☐ Bedrest with bathroom privileges
- ☐ Out of Bed to chair
- ☐ Out of Bed to chair for meals
- ☐ Ambulate with assistance
- ☐ Up Ad Lib

Laboratory
- ☑ Clostridium difficile Antigen/Toxin Screen - If diarrhea persists greater than 72 hours

Patient Care
- ☑ Ramsay Scale - Routine - Assess sedation level using Ramsay or RASS sedation scale. If patient responds to verbal stimulus, AND is less than Ramsay 5 or greater than or equal to RASS -3, proceed with CAM-ICU delirium assessment.
- ☑ Confusion Assessment Method (CAM) - Routine - every shift and PRN. If patient responds to verbal stimulus, AND is less than Ramsay 5 or greater than or equal to RASS -3, proceed with CAM-ICU delirium assessment OR Perform if patient develops acute mental status change
- ☑ Provider to RN Notification - Routine - If skin breakdown present or develops, obtain order for rectal tube unless contraindicated
- ☑ Provider to RN Notification - Routine - Assess need for pain control and anxiety medication and consult ordering clinician as appropriate. Assess need for lines, tubes, restraints daily.
- ☑ Provider to RN Notification - Routine - Promote day/night orientation -Shades open/lights on during daytime -Shades closed/lights off at night - Re-orient patient frequently to date, time, location -Reduce excessive noise stimuli in and around patient room -Promote night time uninterrupted sleep as patient condition permits
- ☑ Provider to RN Notification - Routine - Ensure patient has dentures, hearing aid, glasses if applicable

Notify Physician
- ☑ Notify Physician if no bowel movement by ICU day 5

Medications - Anxiolytics/Sedatives
- ▸ **Avoid benzodiazepines (LORazepam, diazepam, ALPRAZolam, midazolam) and diphenhydrAMINE for sedation and sleep**
- ▸ **Consider discontinuing and minimizing benzodiazepine and anti-histaminic medications**
- ▸ **Review Universal Medication List (UML) and restart home psychotropic medications if appropriate**
- ☐ QUEtiapine. (SERAQUEL) 25 mg by mouth every 6 hours as needed for mild agitation/anxiety to achieve Ramsay score of 2 to 3 or RASS score of -2 to -3. PRN
- ☐ QUEtiapine. (SERAQUEL) 25 mg by nasogastric tube every 6 hours as needed for mild agitation/anxiety to achieve Ramsay score of 2 to 3 or RASS score of -2 to -3. PRN
- ☐ QUEtiapine. (SERAQUEL) 50 mg by mouth every 12 hours as needed for moderate agitation/anxiety to achieve Ramsay score of 2 to 3 or RASS score of -2 to -3. PRN
- ☐ QUEtiapine. (SERAQUEL) 50 mg by nasogastric tube every 12 hours as needed for moderate agitation/anxiety to achieve Ramsay score of 2 to 3 or RASS score of -2 to -3. PRN
- ☐ haloperidol inj (HALDOL) 2 mg IV Push every 2 hours as needed for mild agitation/anxiety to achieve Ramsay score of 2 to 3 or RASS score of -2 to -3. * Notify Physician if prolonged QTc (greater than 500 milliseconds) on EKG. Do not exceed 30 mg in 24 hour period.
- ☐ haloperidol inj (HALDOL) 5 mg IV Push every 2 hours as needed for moderate agitation/anxiety to achieve Ramsay score of 2 to 3 or RASS score of -2 to -3. * Notify Physician if prolonged QTc (greater than 500 milliseconds) on EKG. Do not exceed 30 mg in 24 hour period.
- ☐ haloperidol inj (HALDOL) 10 mg IV Push every 2 hours as needed for severe agitation/anxiety to achieve Ramsay score of 2 to 3 or RASS score of -2 to -3. Stop after 2 doses. * Notify Physician if prolonged QTc (greater than 500 milliseconds) on EKG. Do not exceed 30 mg in 24 hour period.

Physician Signature:_____Provider # _____   Date_____   Time_____

(Rev. 01/21/13) Delirium
ICU Order Set PHYSICIAN
ORDERS
Page 1 of 2

Fig. 1. ICU delirium order set. (*Courtesy of* Baylor Health Care System. Copyright ©2013.)

PHYSICIAN ORDERS

Medications - Other

☑ senna/docusate sodium. (SENNA-S) 1 tablet by mouth 2 times daily.

☑ senna/docusate sodium. (SENNA-S) 1 tablet by nasogastric tube 2 times daily.

☑ bisacodyl enteric coated (DULCOLAX) 10 mg by mouth 1 time daily.Hold if greater than 2 bowel movements in 24 hours or liquid stool greater than 300 mL. When without diarrhea for 48 hours, resume Bisacodyl per daily bowel maintenance program.

☑ bisacodyl suppository (DULCOLAX) 10 mg rectally 1 time daily. Hold if greater than 2 bowel movements in 24 hours or liquid stool greater than 300 mL. When without diarrhea for 48 hours, resume Bisacodyl per daily bowel maintenance program.

☑ magnesium citrate. 150 mL by mouth, 1 time daily as needed for constipation. Start if no bowel movement by ICU day 3. Hold if greater than 4 bowel movements in 24 hours or liquid stool greater than 300 mL. If no response in 24 hours repeat dose. PRN

☑ magnesium citrate. 150 mL by nasogastric tube, 1 time daily as needed for constipation. Start if no bowel movement by ICU day 3. Hold if greater than 4 bowel movements in 24 hours or liquid stool greater than 300 mL. If no response in 24 hours repeat dose. PRN

☑ polyethylene glycol 3350 (MIRALAX) 17 g by mouth 2 times daily as needed for constipation. Start if no bowel movement by ICU day 4. Hold if greater than 4 bowel movements in 24 hours or liquid stool greater than 300 mL. PRN

☑ polyethylene glycol 3350 (MIRALAX) 17 g by nasogastric tube 2 times daily as needed for constipation. Start if no bowel movement by ICU day 4. Hold if greater than 4 bowel movements in 24 hours or liquid stool greater than 300 mL. PRN

☐ dexmedetomidine drip 200 mcg 0.2 mcg/kg/hr. Titrate to maintain Ramsay Sedation Score equal to 2 to 3. Initiate for severe agitation not controlled by quetiapine and haloperidol. * Titrate by 0.1 mcg/kg/hour every 20 minutes to achieve Ramsay score 2 to 3 or RASS score of -2 to -3. This is a starting rate only. Please refer to FLOW SHEET for the most current rate for this titrateable drip.

Department Referrals

☑ Evaluate and Treat Physical Therapy

☑ Evaluate and Treat Occupational Therapy

☑ Pharmacy Consult Request

Saline Flush

☑ sodium chloride 0.9% flush (lock flush)

Physician Signature:_____Provider # _____   Date_____   Time_____

(Rev. 01/21/13) Delirium ICU Order Set PHYSICIAN ORDERS Page 2 of 2

Fig. 1. (*continued*)

CASE STUDY 2

The Society of Critical Care Medicine (SCCM) has developed clinical practice guidelines for managing pain, agitation, and delirium in patients in the ICU. It recommends medications to use for delirious patients and those experiencing pain. This case study discusses a patient in the MICU whose delirium, agitation, and pain were difficult to control. It compares this patient's particular care with the newest SCCM guidelines and shows that even with education and a delirium screening tool in place, management may remain difficult.

Ms H., a 44-year-old woman, was transported to the Emergency Department from home by Emergency Medical Services for shortness of breath and decreased mental status. She was subsequently admitted to the MICU with a diagnosis of shortness of breath and encephalopathy. According to her accompanying fiancé, her home BiPAP machine had broken a few days before admission. Her medical history includes hypertension, chronic obstructive pulmonary disease, tobacco abuse, migraine headaches, asthma, and obesity.

She arrived to the MICU intubated and mechanically ventilated. Her Ramsey scale score was 5 on admission. A CAM-ICU and a Ramsey score were assessed and documented once each shift throughout her hospitalization. In this way, her risk for delirium and her sedation level were closely monitored. Within 12 hours of admission to the MICU, Ms H. began to demonstrate symptoms of hyperactive delirium. Hyperactive delirium often includes delusions, hallucinations, and hyperactivity.[23] Because of her inability to communicate verbally due to an endotracheal tube, it was difficult to determine if Ms H. suffered from delusions and hallucinations. She was CAM-ICU-positive and her agitation was very difficult to control, so a propofol infusion was initiated, but was not completely effective. While on it, she pulled on her tubes and lines and attempted to exit the bed. The SCCM Clinical Practice Guidelines recommend light versus deep levels of sedation.[24] However, because of her hyperactive delirium, Ms H. required a deeper level of sedation. Nonrestraining mittens were applied to both hands. These mittens were not tied to the bed frame as a typical restraint would be; they were wrapped around the hands, leaving the fingertips exposed, thereby allowing only gross movement of the hands. Ms H. was then unable to grab hold of lines and tubes, preventing their removal. Interestingly, Ms H. was taking paroxetine, an antidepressant, before admission. It was not restarted until 2 weeks after she was admitted. It could be possible that she experienced discontinuation syndrome.

Early mobility is recommended to prevent delirium in ICU patients.[24] Because of her agitation and constant movement, Ms H. was essentially performing active range of motion. Her activity level was not able to be increased because of her inability to cooperate and her obesity. She was unable to dangle, sit on the edge of the bed, or walk while she was delirious.

Traditionally, nurses are taught ways to prevent or minimize confusion in geriatric patients. The same prevention measures apply to delirious patients as well,[23] yet it can be difficult to implement these tactics in a large ICU. The guidelines recommend keeping noise at a minimum and allowing for extended periods of uninterrupted sleep[24]; however, the ICU environment by nature is noisy. Although this unit dims lights at night, some lights remain on out of necessity to visualize patients.

The facility's delirium order set was implemented 5 days after Ms H.'s admission (see **Fig. 1**). Before that, individual delirium prevention orders were written at the medical team's discretion. Haloperidol intravenous push was used with limited success. Use of haloperidol is not supported by the SCCM, because there is no evidence that haloperidol is useful in delirious patients in the ICU.[24] A dexmedetomidine infusion was also initiated in conjunction with the propofol infusion started quickly after admission. These medications together were still not effective in controlling the patient's agitation and delirium, so an infusion of midazolam was started along with the propofol and dexmedetomidine infusions. Benzodiazepines such as midazolam are widely known to cause delirium, and every attempt to avoid its use was made in Ms H.'s case. Midazolam is not a preferred medication because of its long half-life of 3 to 11 hours. This half-life makes sedation vacations and spontaneous breathing trials less frequent and more difficult to perform. Getting the patient to wake up and breathe is vital to ventilator weaning and extubation. Quetiapine 50 mg per nasogastric tube every 8 hours was started within 2 days of admission. Over a period of days, this helped Ms H. become calmer. She eventually responded to commands appropriately and was CAM-ICU-negative. At that time, the patient was weaned off of midazolam, propofol, and dexmedetomidine. Quetiapine was later decreased to 50 mg daily because of excessive sleepiness. Ms H. was alert and oriented by ICU day 13. Fentanyl IV pushes were used to control her discomfort.

Ms H. failed all attempts to wean from the ventilator during her stay. She received a tracheotomy 12 days after admission. She had a CAM-ICU-positive score most of her stay, with the exception the last week of her hospitalization.

Ms H. was discharged to a long-term care facility after a 27-day hospital stay. She was CAM-ICU-negative on discharge. She was alert, oriented to time, place, and person, and followed commands appropriately.

IMPLICATIONS FOR NURSING PRACTICE

Take into account the knowledge base of the nurses, physicians, and therapy team, as well as the patient's behavior and diagnosis, and delirium prevention, incidence, and treatment in the ICU setting can be a complex adaptive system in itself. Hard-wired processes need to be in place to detect and treat delirium as quickly as possible. Nursing staff is in the forefront of this process, because nurses are the key stakeholders in screening for evidence of delirium and making sure nonpharmacological prevention measures are in place.

REFERENCES

1. Merriam-Webster dictionary. Delirium. Merriam-Webster dictionary. Available at: www.merriam-webster.com. Accessed November 15, 2013.
2. Arend E, Christensen M. Delirium in the intensive care unit: a review. Nurs Crit Care 2009;14:145–54.
3. Lipowski ZJ. Delirium in the elderly patient. N Engl J Med 1989;320:578–82.
4. Trzepacz PT. The neuropathogenesis of delirium: a need to focus our research. Psychosomatics 1994;35:374–91.
5. Smith MJ, Breitbart WS, Platt MM. A critique of instruments and methods to detect, diagnose, and rate delirium. J Pain Symptom Manage 1995;10:35–77.
6. Jacobson S, Schreibman B. Behavioral and pharmacologic treatment of delirium. Am Fam Physician 1997;56:2005–12.
7. Rummans TA, Evans JM, Krahn LE, et al. Delirium in elderly patients: evaluation and management. Mayo Clin Proc 1995;70:989–98.
8. Mach JR, Kabet V, Olson D, et al. Delirium and right-hemisphere dysfunction in cognitively impaired older persons. Int Psychogeriatr 1996;8:373–82.
9. Rudberg MA, Pompei P, Foreman MD, et al. The natural history of delirium in older hospitalized patients: a syndrome of heterogeneity. Age Ageing 1997; 26:169–74.
10. Lin S, Huang C, Liu C, et al. Risk factors for the development of early-onset delirium and the subsequent clinical outcome in mechanically ventilated patients. J Crit Care 2008;23:372–9.
11. Ely EW, Shintani A, Truman B, et al. Delirium as a predictor of mortality in mechanically ventilated patients in the intensive care unit. JAMA 2004; 291(14):1753–62.
12. Van Rompaey B, Schuurmans MJ, Shortridge-Baggett LM, et al. Long term outcome after delirium in the intensive care unit. J Clin Nurs 2009;18(23):3349–57.
13. Pisani MA, Kong SY, Kael SV, et al. Days of delirium are associated with a 1-year mortality in older intensive care unit population. Am J Respir Crit Care Med 2009; 180(11):1092–7.
14. Gottesman RF, Grega MA, Bailey MM, et al. Delirium after coronary artery bypass graft surgery and late mortality. Ann Neurol 2010;67(3):338–44.
15. Stuck A, Clark MJ, Connelly C. Preventing intensive care unit delirium a patient-centered approach to reducing sleep disruption. Dimens Crit Care Nurs 2011; 30(6):315–20.
16. Jackson JC, Gordon SM, Hart RP, et al. The association between delirium and cognitive decline: a review of the empirical literature. Neuropsychol Rev 2004; 14(2):87–98.
17. Milbrandt EB, Deppen S, Harrison PL, et al. Costs associated with delirium in mechanically ventilated patients. Crit Care Med 2004;32(4):955–62.
18. Leslie DL, Marcantonio ER, Zhang Y, et al. One-year health care costs associated with delirium in the elderly population. Arch Intern Med 2008;168(1):27–32.
19. Eeles EMP, Hubbard RE, White SV, et al. Hospital use, institutionalization and mortality associated with delirium. Age Ageing 2010;39:470–5.

20. Inouye SK, Bogardus ST Jr, Charpentier PA, et al. A multi-component intervention to prevent delirium in hospitalized older patients. N Engl J Med 1999;340(9): 669–76.
21. Milisen K, Foreman MD, Abraham IL, et al. A nurse-led interdisciplinary intervention program for delirium in elderly hip-fracture patients. J Am Geriatr Soc 2001; 49(5):523–32.
22. Robinson S, Rich C, Weitzel T, et al. Delirium prevention for cognitive, sensory, and mobility impairments. Res Theory Nurs Pract 2008;22(2):103–13.
23. Balas MC, Rice M, Chaperon C, et al. Management of delirium in critically ill older adults. Crit Care Nurse 2012;32(4):15–26.
24. Barr J, Fraser GL, Puntillo K, et al. Clinical practice guidelines for the management of pain, agitation, and delirium in adult patients in the intensive care unit. Crit Care Med 2013;41(1):263–306.

Stroke Care Using a Hub and Spoke Model with Telemedicine

Penny Huddleston, PhD(c), RN, CCRN[a],*,
Mary Beth Zimmermann, MSN, RN, ACNS-BC[b]

KEYWORDS

- Stroke • Telemedicine • Tissue plaminogen activator • Hub • Spoke

KEY POINTS

- The hub and spoke model provides access to specialty care in hospitals.
- Telemedicine provides neurology expertise to patients requiring stroke care.
- The use of tissue plaminogen activator improves outcomes for patients who have been diagnosed with an ischemic stroke.
- Early detection of a stroke saves lives.

Currently, stroke is the fourth leading cause of death in the United States; these deaths account for approximately 130,000 deaths annually or 1 in every 19 deaths.[1] More than 795,000 people in the United States will have a stroke each year, with 610,000 people having a new stroke and 185,000 people having recurrent strokes.[2] Ischemic strokes account for 87% of all strokes; of the remaining strokes, 10% are intracerebral hemorrhages, and 3% are subarachnoid hemorrhages.[2] On average, a person has a stroke every 40 seconds in the United States. The estimated cost for direct and indirect stroke care is $73.7 billion each year in the United States alone.[2] Stroke is the leading cause of serious long-term disability.[2] With the prevalence and significance of this disease process, the American Heart Association and the American Stroke Association (AHA/ASA) have challenged health care workers to provide evidence-based care that is timely to this patient population.

PROBLEM STATEMENT

Recommendations from the AHA/ASA have resulted in patients with stroke-like symptoms being taken to a primary stroke center (PSC) or comprehensive stroke center

Disclosure Statement: The authors have no disclosures to claim.
[a] Department of Administration, Baylor Medical Center at Irving, 1901 N. MacArthur Boulevard, Irving, TX 75061, USA; [b] Department of Stroke Administration, Texas Health Harris Methodist Fort Worth, 1301 Pennsylvania Avenue, Fort Worth, TX 76104, USA
* Corresponding author.
E-mail address: PennyHu@BaylorHealth.edu

(CSC) to receive evidence-based care.[2] Emergency medical service (EMS) programs have been trained to alert centers to activate their stroke teams to be prepared to care for patients with stroke-like symptoms to save minutes and brain cells.[3] Earlier treatment in patients with stroke-like symptoms can be significant by preventing delays in appropriate therapies, such as recombinant tissue plasminogen activator (rt-PA), which may result in reversal of these symptoms.[4] Poorer outcomes with increased brain tissue damage may occur with delays in delivering appropriate therapy.[4] Fifteen percent to 40% of patients with symptoms of an acute stroke will arrive at hospitals early enough to receive thrombolytic therapy, while only 2% to 5% of these patients actually will receive rt-PA.[5]

Treatment gaps for patients diagnosed with a stroke include the availability of physicians who specialize in stroke care and timely access to evidence-based stroke care.[6] Telemedicine for patients with stroke-like symptoms, or Telestroke, was developed in 1999 using video telecommunications.[6] Telestroke has assisted in bridging this gap to provide effective stroke treatment to patients with their treatment location or when the time required to evaluate patients by a specialist in the emergency department may be a barrier preventing access to appropriate stroke care. The purpose of this article is to describe how the implementation of a hub and spoke model using telemedicine in a large health care system in the United States has assisted in closing this gap by increasing patient access to neurology expertise and the patient receiving evidence-based treatment, thereby improving patient outcomes.

REVIEW OF THE LITERATURE

The AHA/ASA published recommendations for evidence-based stroke care that includes:

- Importance of becoming a PCS or CSC
- Response time of the stroke team in less than 15 minutes
- Initiation of telemedicine link within 20 minutes of arrival of the patient to the emergency department
- Computerized tomography (CT)/laboratory/chest radiograph/electrocardiography results in less than 45 minutes
- Door to rt-PA of less than 60 minutes in those patients with symptom onset up to 3 and recently out to 4.5 hours
- Neurosurgery consultation within 2 hours of emergency department arrival time
- Bedside swallow screen
- Patient education
- EMS guidelines with recommendations to take patients to a PSC or CSC
- Public education on when to seek medical care
- Drug therapy for stroke care
- Radiographic guidelines for stroke care
- Surgical interventions[2,3,7]

These recommendations are part of the standardized criteria set forth by The Joint Commission (TJC) for PSCs and CSCs to ensure the best outcomes for patients with stroke-like symptoms.

The published literature outlines the significance of using telemedicine to provide evidence-based stroke care. The use of telemedicine is an innovative method to bridge the gap between access to care and the availability of neurology expertise. Telemedicine provides early access to remote specialist assessment, real-time clinical evaluation and interpretation of brain imaging, and evidence-based treatment using thrombolysis for acute ischemic strokes.[6,8]

A systematic review of the literature showed that over 20 studies (cross-sectional, longitudinal, and randomized controlled trials) have been conducted since 2002.[6] Most studies focused on the proportions of patients with stroke symptoms receiving rt-PA and the time it took to deliver this treatment. Retrospective and prospective studies showed that using telemedicine for remote consultation and delivery of a thrombolytic agent was feasible without additional risk to the patient.[6–8] Multiple research studies demonstrated that Telestroke care was as safe as on-site stroke care, while the hub and spoke model also improved patient outcomes resulting from neurology expertise.[4–6,8–11] Correct treatment decisions using telemedicine occurred 98% of the time in the telemedicine group and 82% in the telephonic group, with a P value of .0009.[6] There was no statistical difference in 90-day functional capacity, mortality, or rate of intracerebral hemorrhage after treatment with rt-PA was found between the 2 groups. In these studies, no consultations were aborted; however, technical difficulties occurred 74% of the time.[6] The technical difficulties did not prevent correct treatment decisions but did affect the time to treatment.

According to 20 studies conducted between 2003 and 2010, 15,000 patients presented to acute care hospital facilities with acute stroke symptoms.[6] In the earlier studies, the review of literature showed that telemedical management of acute stroke was safe, feasible, and acceptable, while in recent studies, the randomized controlled trials confirmed the effectiveness of the use of telemedicine to bridge the gap in reducing the geographic differences by improving accessibility to evidence-based care, increasing diagnostic accuracy, and increasing thrombolytic treatment.[6] These studies did show an increase in the evaluation time by telemedicine and an increase in technical difficulties.[6–8]

IMPLEMENTATION OF THE HUB AND SPOKE MODEL

A team of doctors and nurses met to discuss the possibility of implementing a hub and spoke model at a large urban health care system in the Dallas/Fort Worth area. The goal was to provide evidence-based stroke care by improving access to care, decreasing the time to receive care, and decreasing the number of patients transferred to the larger health care facility. A largest hospital in the health care system functioned as the hub hospital, while other hospitals within the health care system functioned as the spoke hospitals. In January 2013 the hub and spoke model using telemedicine for stroke care was implemented with one of the smaller hospitals being the first to embark on becoming a spoke hospital. Guidelines were agreed upon between the hub and spoke hospitals (**Fig. 1**). The staff was educated and demonstrated competency on evidence-based stroke care. The staff was also educated on the process of when to activate a code stroke and when to call the hub hospital to alert the neurologist on-call of the patient's arrival to the spoke hospital. The hub and spoke hospitals practiced mock code stroke calls to address any areas of concern.

Physicians and nurses assess the patient using the National Institutes of Health Stroke Scale (NIHSS) and obtain a computerized tomography scan, a chest radiograph, laboratory tests, and an electrocardiography examination as quickly as possible. The technician pages the neuro-hospitalist on-call at the hub hospital. The neuro-hospitalist consults with the emergency department physician to determine the appropriate treatment for the patient based on the diagnosis.

Stroke Hub and Spoke Model Flowchart

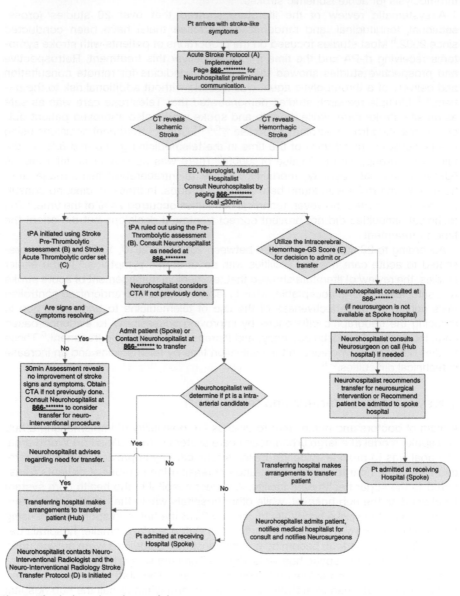

Fig. 1. The hub and spoke model.

Once the treatment is determined, the emergency department physician implements the treatment. At eight o'clock the following morning, the neuro-hospitalist from the spoke hospital takes over the care of the patient from the hub neuro-hospitalist.

CASE STUDY

In August 2013, a 64-year-old woman with a history of hypertension and smoking developed sudden onset of left facial droop and weakness of the left upper and left lower extremities while attempting to make her grocery list one Saturday morning. She was last seen normal without symptoms at 9:45 AM. The patient's husband rushed her to the spoke hospital emergency department where the triage nurse quickly recognized the signs and symptoms of a possible cerebral vascular accident (CVA) and notified the charge nurse and emergency department physician. The patient's arrival time was 10:28 AM. The NIHSS was performed by the emergency department physician and was noted to be a score of 12. The patient promptly received a CT scan of the brain. The emergency department physician reviewed the results at 11:22 AM. The chest radiograph was ordered with the results back to the ED physician at 11:12 AM. The emergency department physician reviewed the electrocardiography at 11:01 AM and the laboratory tests at 11:12 AM. All results were normal.

The emergency department physician implemented the stroke protocol for the hub and spoke model, by contacting the neuro-hospitalist at the spoke hospital at the 10:55 AM. The nurse in the emergency department properly positioned the robot in front of the patient to be utilized by the neuro-hospitalist. The patient was interviewed and examined by a physician at hub hospital via an electronic tablet with real-time audiovisual capabilities. During the examination by the neuro-hospitalist, the patient was noted to have left-sided weakness, left facial droop, and dysarthria with an NIHSS of 9. The CT scan of the head was reviewed via the PACS interface on an electronic tablet by the neuro-hospitalist including revealed no hemorrhage. The treatment intervention and the risks and benefits of intravenous t-PA were discussed with the family, and it was noted she had no contraindications to thrombolysis. The patient received rt-PA 0.9 mg/kg at 11:42 AM. The patient's symptoms began to improve, and the physicians determined that did not need to be transferred the patient to the hub hospital. The patient was admitted to the spoke hospital's stroke unit and was transferred to inpatient rehabilitation after 5 days. The patient was discharged from the inpatient rehabilitation unit 10 days after the initial emergency department visit. Today, the patient has some residual left-sided weakness, but it is improving on a daily basis. Without the hub and spoke model and telemedicine, the patient would have been transferred to another local hospital, where a delay in receiving evidence-based care could have impacted the patient outcome.

DISCUSSION

As a result of the implementation of the hub and spoke model with telemedicine, this spoke hospital has become a PCS-certified hospital and is able to maintain core at measures greater than the 80th percentile. This model has improved access to care, increased availability of neurology expertise, increased the number of patients receiving rt-PA, and decreased the number of adverse events in patients diagnosed with a stroke in this spoke facility. Without the hub and spoke model with telemedicine at rural or community-based hospitals that do not have access to timely neurologic expertise, patients may not receive evidence-based stroke care in a timely and efficient manner.

LINKAGE TO THE COMPLEX ADAPTIVE SYSTEM

A complex adaptive system (CAS) is defined as individual elements that may have unpredictable actions, which are interconnected so that one element's actions may change the context of the other elements.[12] Characteristics of a CAS include the following:

- Elements interacting in a dynamic manner with an exchange of information
- Interactions that are rich and non-linear, with a limited range as a result of no framework to control the flow of information

- Feedback loops that may be positive or negative
- Continual changes that result in the flow of energy into the system
- Functions independently with no historical knowledge of actions, but the effects operate within the system
- Patterns of interactions between the elements[12]

The implementation of a hub and spoke model with telemedicine for acute stroke care is an example of a CAS.

A large heath care system implemented a hub and spoke model with a telemedicine to better meet the needs of patients diagnosed with stroke. The spoke hospitals function in concert with the hub hospital in a dynamic manner with the sharing of information from hospitals. Interactions between the spoke hospitals and the hub hospital are rich using telemedicine as it results in nonlinear communication based on the individual conditions of the patients with stroke-like symptoms and the specialty services each hospital provides in relationship to stroke care. Feedback loops between the hub hospital and spoke hospitals assist in the overall interactions and patterns of the CAS. The hub and spoke model with telemedicine is dynamic, with similar patterns set forth by the evidence-based practice guidelines, but no one spoke hospital functions the same as another spoke hospital based on the specialty services available. Continual changes occur within these processes using best practices that result in access to care with neurology consultation and the best outcomes for patients receiving stroke care.

IMPLICATIONS FOR PRACTICE

The development of the hub and spoke model with telemedicine for stroke care offers opportunities to provide stroke treatment in rural areas or areas where 24-hour coverage of neurologic specialists such as neuro-hospitalists or stroke neurologists is unavailable. This hub and spoke model also allows improving the quality of care for acute stroke patients by improving access to care, decreasing door-to-needle time, increasing the number of patients treated with rt-PA, and reducing the reluctance of emergency department physicians to give the drug. This method improves access to physicians so time-sensitive therapies can be administered.[9]

The hub and spoke model increases the number of patients being treated with rt-PA. This, combined with telemedicine expertise, can increase the number of patients treated with rt-PA in community hospitals.[10] Telemedicine decreases the number of transfers to the hub hospital allowing patients to stay close to their community and family.[11] Telemedicine also allows identification of those patients who require transfer to a hub facility for surgery or interventional procedures, such as patients with hemorrhage or basilar artery occlusions.[11]

Since implementation of the hub and spoke model, this service has been consulted 239 times from January 2013 to July 2014. Of those consultations, 37 out of 39 patients were deemed eligible for rt-PA treatment. Two hundred and twenty-seven patients were kept at the spoke hospital after consultation and 12 patients required transfer to the hub hospital. Prior to the implementation of the hub and spoke model for stroke at this hospital, only one patient was treated with intravenous rt-PA (**Box 1**).

Several barriers to intravenous rt-PA treatment exist despite the evidence that shows benefit from receiving this drug within three hours of stroke-like symptoms onset. Only 2% to 5% of these patients actually receive rt-PA.[5] This can be attributed to several factors including:

- A physician's lack of familiarity or inexperience giving the drug
- A decrease in the availability of neurology expertise

Box 1	
Implementation of the hub and spoke model	
January 2013 Through July 2014	
No. of patients eligible for intravenous rtPA	39
No. of patients who received intravenous rtPA	37
% Patients who received intravenous rtPA	94.87%
Total number of hub and spoke patients	239

Telemedicine can fill the gap needed to address these issues. In addition, telemedicine may also lead to earlier diagnosis of patients who need to transfer to a hub hospital, including those with subarachnoid hemorrhage or intracranial hemorrhage patients who require surgical intervention.[11]

REFERENCES

1. Centers for Disease Control and Prevention. Stroke facts. Atlanta, Georgia: Centers for Disease Control and Prevention; 2013. Available at: http://www.cdc.gov.
2. Go AS, Mozaffarian D, Roger VL, et al. Heart disease and stroke statistics—2013 update: a report from the American Heart Association. Circulation 2013;127: e6–245. http://dx.doi.org/10.1161/CIR.0b013e31828124ad.
3. Jauch EC, Saver JL, Adams HP, et al. Guidelines for early management of patients with acute ischemic stroke: a guideline for healthcare professionals from the American Heart Association/American Stroke Association. Stroke 2013;44: 870–947. http://dx.doi.org/10.1161/STR.0b013e318284056a.
4. Meyers BC, Raman R, Ernstrom K, et al. Assessment of long-term outcomes for the STRokE DOC telemedicine trial. J Stroke Cerebrovasc Dis 2012;21:259–64. http://dx.doi.org/10.1016/j.jstrokecerebrovasdis.2010.08.004.
5. Walter S, Kostopoulos P, Haass A, et al. Diagnosis and treatment of patients with stroke in a mobile stroke unit versus in hospital: a randomized controlled trial. Lancet 2012;11:397–404. http://dx.doi.org/10.1016/S1474-4422(12)70057-1.
6. Roots A, Bhalla A, Birns J. Telemedicine for stroke: a systematic review. Br J Neurosci Nurs 2011;7:481–9.
7. Albert MJ, Wechsler LR, Lee-Jensen ME, et al. Formation and function of acute stroke-ready hospitals within a stroke system of care recommendations from the brain attack coalition. Stroke 2013;44:1–15. http://dx.doi.org/10.1161/STROKEAHA.113.002285.
8. Birns J. Innovations in the assessment and management of stroke: the use of telemedicine. Br J Neurosci Nurs 2010;6:66–9. Available at: http://www.bjnn.co.uk.
9. Hess DC, Wang S, Gross H, et al. Telestroke: extending stroke expertise into underserved areas. Lancet 2006;5:275–8. http://dx.doi.org/10.1016/S1474-4422(06) 70377-5.
10. Schwamm LH, Holloway RG, Amarenco P, et al. A review of the evidence for the use of telemedicine within stroke systems of care: a scientific statement from the American Heart Association/American Stroke Association. Stroke 2009;40: 2616–34. http://dx.doi.org/10.1161/STROKE/AHA.109.192360.
11. Tatlisumak TS, Soinila S, Kaste M. Telestroke networking offers multiple benefits beyond thrombolysis. Cerebrovasc Dis 2009;27:21–7. http://dx.doi.org/10.1159/000213055.
12. Holden LM. Complex adaptive systems: concept analysis. J Adv Nurs 2005;52: 651–7. http://dx.doi.org/10.1111/j.1365-2648.2005.03638.x.

Application of a Robot for Critical Care Rounding in Small Rural Hospitals

Cindy Murray, MBA, MHA, BSN, RN, CENP, CNOR[a],*,
Elizabeth Ortiz, MBA, BSN, RN, NEA-BC[b], Cay Kubin, BSN, RN, CNML[c]

KEYWORDS

- Critical care rounding • Remote presence robot • Critical care physician shortage
- Faster access and improved quality and finance outcomes • Stroke care
- Telemedicine

KEY POINTS

- There is a national shortage of critical care and specialty physicians.
- Critical care physicians can round on patients in intensive care units via a remote presence robot from their offices or other setting.
- Small rural hospitals can realize improvements in quality and finance metrics using a remote presence robot model by bringing critical care physicians to patients.
- The patient care team can benefit from additional education provided by specialists.
- Use of a remote presence robot can be expanded beyond the walls of the intensive care unit, for example, in the emergency department for the care of patients who have had a stroke.

INTRODUCTION

Baylor Medical Center at Waxahachie (BMCW) is a licensed 69 bed acute care facility located approximately 30 miles south of Dallas, Texas. BMCW serves all of Ellis County as well as outlying areas, covering a population of roughly 150,000. As a small hospital in a somewhat rural setting, BMCW has struggled in the past to provide continuous specialty physician coverage to the patients in the intensive care unit (ICU).

Disclosures: None applicable.
[a] Department of Administration, Baylor Medical Center at Waxahachie, 1405 West Jefferson, Waxahachie, TX 75165, USA; [b] Acute Care Services, Baylor Medical Center at Waxahachie, 1405 West Jefferson, Waxahachie, TX 75165, USA; [c] Intensive Care Unit, Baylor Medical Center at Waxahachie, 1405 West Jefferson, Waxahachie, TX 75165, USA
* Corresponding author.
E-mail address: Cindymur@baylorhealth.edu

Crit Care Nurs Clin N Am 26 (2014) 477–485
http://dx.doi.org/10.1016/j.ccell.2014.08.006
0899-5885/14/$ – see front matter © 2014 Elsevier Inc. All rights reserved.

ccnursing.theclinics.com

With a national shortage of critical care physicians, BMCW was challenged with recruiting the needed number of specialists to cover its critical care patient population.[1] The health care climate was changing, and various models of physician care were being introduced nationally to improve access, quality, and decrease cost. The message from the community was also clear: there was a strong desire to not have loved ones transferred out of the local hospital. BMCW needed a way to meet those challenges. So in 2008, BMCW began researching alternate methods of covering their sickest, frailest patients, from ramping up recruitment efforts to ICU coverage.

THE SOLUTION

Meet Baylor's Extra Specialist Seeing You (BESSY), a remote presence robot that allows a physician miles away to interact with patients via a 2-way audio/video robot.[2] This robot, similar in appearance to Rosie the cartoon character from the Jetsons (**Fig. 1**), supports real-time communication between the specialty physician, patient, and other care team members. Unlike Skype (Skype Technologies, S.A., Luxembourg City, Luxembourg), there is no delay in the communication via the remote presence robot. This innovative technology ensures that the physician from the remote location can use a laptop and joystick to control the robot at the facility. The physician directs the robot around the ICU to make rounds. The technology allows the remote physician to view the patient care monitors and ventilator settings; listen to heart/lung sounds; examine pupils; and interact with patients, family members, and/or the care team.

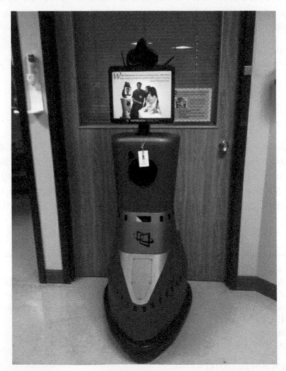

Fig. 1. BESSY: a remote presence robot that allows a physician miles away to interact with patients via a 2-way audio/video robot.

The benefits of telemedicine include faster access to specialists, increased convenience for patients and families, improved equity of access to care between regions, and improved quality of care.[3] Using this innovative technology, BMCW has been able to bring medical specialists from Baylor University Medical Center (BUMC) in Dallas, some 30 miles away, to the patients' bedside within moments. The critical care consulting physicians are brought to the bedside via BESSY as members of the health care team at a moment's notice 24 hours a day, 7 days a week. This model involves the on-site hospitalists and remote critical care specialists rounding daily and comanaging critical care patients.

FASTER ACCESS, IMPROVED FINANCE AND QUALITY OUTCOMES

The remote presence of a specialized physician has made a difference in daily patient care and outcomes for patients at BMCW. There have been several critical situations while BESSY has been part of the team that have necessitated the quick response of a provider with expertise to handle a multisystem failure, high-acuity patients who were too unstable to transfer. These patients required around-the-clock observation and frequent rounding from the intensivist. Had it not been for the pioneering makeup of the health care team, the outcomes achieved would not have been likely. The use of a shared care model is significant in providing optimum care and efficient utilization of resources in BMCW's partnership as a part of the Baylor Health Care System. Using BESSY allows fewer delays in decision making and corresponding actions, saving time for the patients and the health care providers, and provides ongoing educational opportunities.

One hospitalist at our facility notes that, "intensivists are an integral part of managing critically ill patients. The technology of a telemedicine robot offers the intensivists the unique capability to remotely participate in patient care and thus leads to better patient outcomes." In fact, BMCW's own data reflect improved quality for its patients since it began this program in 2008. BMCW's ICU bounce-back rate has been cut in half (**Fig. 2**). Mortality rates have also improved (**Fig. 3**). BMCW has a continued focus

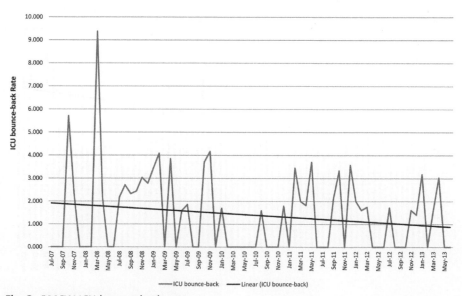

Fig. 2. BMCW ICU bounce-back rate.

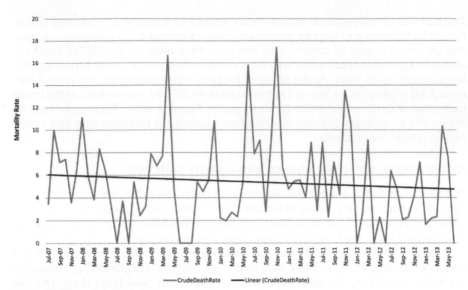

Fig. 3. BMCW mortality rate.

on quality improvement, and the robot serves as a tool for the patient care team to be successful in improving outcomes.

From a financial perspective, BMCW has seen monthly volumes of ICU patients increase by more than 50% (**Fig. 4**), and the average length of stay (LOS) for an ICU patient has improved from an average of 3.3 days to 2.5 days (**Fig. 5**). BMCW has also seen an increase in its case mix index (CMI), ranging from less than 1.20 for this patient population before implementing the robot to greater than 1.40 for current ICU patients (**Fig. 6**). Keeping patients locally allows BMCW to keep the revenue locally and gives a better bottom line.

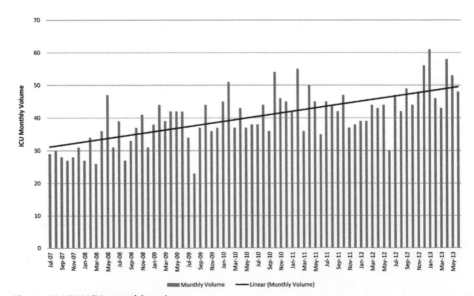

Fig. 4. BMCW ICU monthly volume.

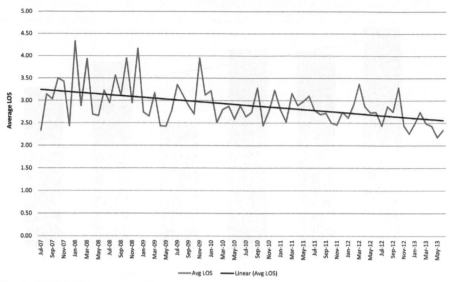

Fig. 5. BMCW ICU average LOS.

CONVENIENCE FOR PATIENTS AND FAMILIES

The families of the patients have expressed satisfaction with their family member remaining in the local hospital. Indeed, BMCW's data reflect that its external transfer rate has declined since implementing this model of care (**Fig. 7**). In addition to staying near home, they are glad that their family is receiving a higher level of care than was possible before this innovative approach to care. Not only do the patients and families benefit from this leading edge technology but also members of the health care team

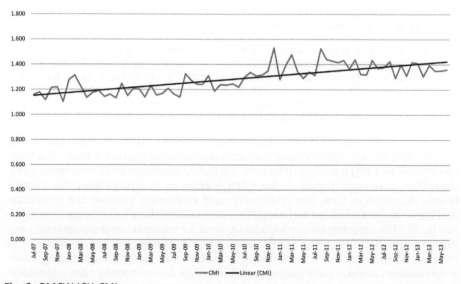

Fig. 6. BMCW ICU CMI.

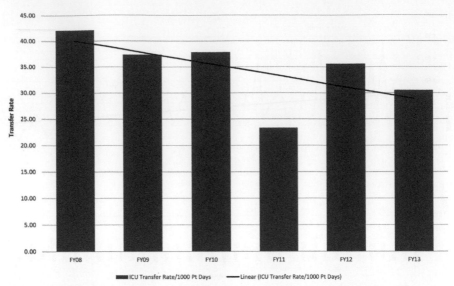

Fig. 7. BMCW transfer from ICU to external facility rate per 1000 patient-days.

have expressed their excitement with the opportunity to be part of such an innovative approach to care.

ACCESS TO CARE BETWEEN REGIONS

The nursing care team has seen a level of care that was once not possible in this small rural hospital. As a direct caregiver, the nurse can round with BESSY and give the physician a report on patients' current conditions. The nurse is still the hands of the physician as BESSY is equipped with a high-definition screen, articulating cameras, stethoscopes, printer, phones, and other instruments that allow the physician to listen and look at physiologic parameters with the assistance of the nurse. One of the critical care nurses has the following to say:

> BESSY, the robot, plays a key role here at Baylor Medical Center at Waxahachie. The benefit of having a specialized ICU physician collaborating with our attending hospitalists results in exceptional care. As a nurse, it's comforting to know that my patients are being cared for through a "second set of eyes," a vital aspect for ICU patients whose condition could change within seconds. It is yet another way Baylor delivers an extraordinary level of care for our patients.

An ICU charge nurse and bedside leader in the ICU notes that the care being provided in this unique way is of higher quality and more time sensitive than in the past. "The robot has been an amazing addition to the team. The BUMC Intensivist and Waxahachie multi-disciplinary care team rounds via the robot enables us to provide the patient with a holistic approach to care. The relationship and confidence between the physicians and the nurses has improved and translates into positive patient outcomes and satisfaction for all." The robot has also provided an avenue for education for the hospitalists and the nursing staff. On more than one occasion, the BUMC intensivist has used BESSY to have impromptu education and mentoring for the care team. In fact, one particular intensivist has been active in participating in staff meetings and presenting case information to educate staff on advanced clinical skills not seen regularly in the rural ICU setting.

INDIVIDUALIZED PATIENT CARE

During the first 6 months of using BESSY and the BUMC intensivists, there was a very ill patient whose level of care could not be provide at BMCW before the deployment of BESSY. This patient would have required immediate transport to BUMC. This story was one of the most dramatic and memorable stories related to the use of BESSY and the effects of teleconsultation. While the team was consulting with the BUMC intensivist via the robot, the patient developed respiratory compromise, which required immediate intubation. The team was able to respond quickly to this emergent need and intubated the patient under the guidance of the intensivist. The patient's respiratory status had been severely compromised, which required high levels of positive end expiratory pressure and oxygen. After two unsuccessful attempts to transfer her to a higher level of care via helicopter because of hemodynamic instability, the intensivist along with the unit care team collaborated on bringing the needed manpower and resources to the patient. One of the complex care needs required to maintain this patient's life was continuous renal replacement therapy. It was critical that this advanced level of care, requiring highly technical skills, be deployed emergently to the bedside in an attempt to stabilize the patient. As a collaborative team, and shared resources within the health care system, the care team could deliver a higher level of care to the bedside, along with the specialized care of the intensivist. This advanced procedure was carried out for approximately 3 days with the guidance of the BUMC intensivist via frequent rounding with the care team using BESSY. Although the resolution of this case was not what the care team would have hoped for, both the staff and family thought everything possible had been attempted, which allowed for an easier transition at the end of life.

STROKE CARE

Because of the success of using BMCW's remote presence robot on critical care patients in the ICU, its emergency department (ED) care team has now partnered with a group of neurologists at BUMC to develop a protocol to use BESSY for providing stroke care for patients presenting in the ED (**Fig. 8**). BMCW sees more than 43,000 patients in its ED annually. Many present with stroke systems. One of BMCW's medical telemetry nurses had the following to say about her family member's experience with neurology specialists using the robot:

At Baylor Waxahachie, I had heard of the 'robot', the name of the rolling telemedicine monitor and it's [sic] usefulness in ICU. It was devised so that specialists in Baylor Dallas could 'see' critically ill patients and treat them quickly without having to waste precious minutes in transfers. Little did I know how important the 'robot' would become to my own family.

On October 3, 2013, my husband collapsed on the front porch after having picked up our daughter from school. He knew something was wrong on the drive home but just brushed it off, thinking it was another one of his migraines. I was at home finalizing preparations for our son's October 5th wedding, when I heard my daughter screaming.

When I reached my husband, I saw him lying there and thought he had somehow tripped and hit his head. I asked him what had happened and he said that his legs went numb. While my daughter dialed 911, I assessed him and he seemed fine until a few moments later. His speech became slurred, the left side of his face drooped, and he stated that he was feeling nauseous. I knew immediately he was having a stroke. I glanced at my watch. It was 4:05 PM.

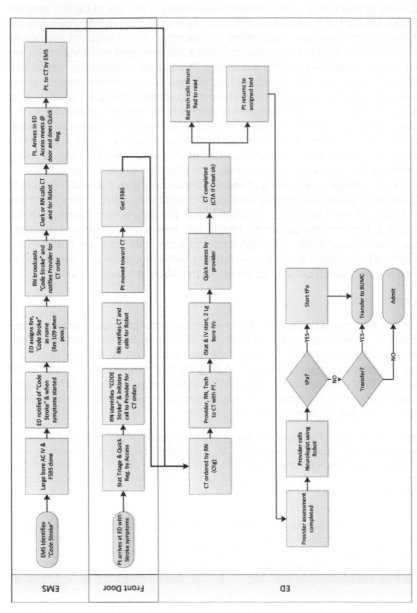

Fig. 8. ED stroke process map. AC, antecubital; Chg, charge; Creat, creatinine; CT, computed tomography; CTA, computed tomography angiogram; EMS, emergency medical services; FSBS, finger stick blood sugar; IStat, name of device used for point of care testing; IV, intravenous; Lg, large; Neuro, neurology; poss, possible; PT and Pt, patient; Rad, radiology; Reg, registration; Rm, room; tech, technician; tPa, tissue plasminogen activator.

The ambulance and firemen arrived quickly and I told them I wanted him taken to Baylor Waxahachie. The [emergency room] ER team worked efficiently in assessing him and getting the necessary CT [computed tomography] and MRI images. It was determined that he had an ischemic stroke and the 'robot' was rolled into the room. On the monitor was a neurologist from Baylor Dallas. After conversing with the ER doctors, studying his images, and virtually 'seeing' my husband, she concluded that he was a candidate for t-PA [tissue plasminogen activator], a clot-busting enzyme given intravenously. If a stroke victim can receive this medicine within three hours of the onset of symptoms, it improves their odds for recovery. I glanced at the clock on the wall - 5:15 PM. He received the t-PA and then transferred via Care Flight to the BUMC's Acute Stroke Unit.

He has made a full recovery and was even able to attend our son's wedding two days later. At his follow up visit, the neurologist stated that after studying his case and looking at his MRI, he was a walking miracle. If he had not received the t-PA, she's certain he would have some residual paralysis on his left side.

Timeliness and efficiency was key in the diagnosing and subsequent treatment of my husband's stroke. The availability of telemedicine was a big part of that process, along with the doctors and nurses. We are so thankful and credit his strong recovery to the great care he received at Baylor Waxahachie.

SUMMARY

Patient care delivery models are changing. Small rural hospitals can improve care to critically ill patients by partnering with specialty physicians to round on patients using a robot. Improvements in quality, finance, patient, and care team satisfaction have been noted.

REFERENCES

1. Angus DC, Shorr AF, White A, et al, on behalf of the Committee on Manpower for Pulmonary and Critical Care Societies (COMPACCS). Critical care delivery in the United States: distribution of services and compliance with Leapfrog recommendations. Crit Care Med 2006;34(4):1016–24.
2. InTouch Health Brochure, Santa Barbara, California.
3. Hjelm N. Benefits and drawbacks of telemedicine. J Telemed Telecare 2005;11(2): 60–70.

Driving Sepsis Mortality Down

Emergency Department and Critical Care Partnerships

Kristine K. Powell, MSN, RN, CEN, NEA-BC[a],*,
Rita J. Fowler, MSN, RN, CCRN, NE-BC[b]

KEYWORDS

- Septicemia • Sepsis • Septic shock • Sepsis mortality • Surviving Sepsis Campaign
- Performance improvement

KEY POINTS

- Sepsis is a complex condition that occurs in the complex systems of the human body.
- Improvements in sepsis care can be difficult in the complex system of health care.
- A continuous quality improvement approach with active engagement of administrative and clinical personnel at all levels is needed to improve sepsis care.
- Rigorous and transparent reporting of metrics based on evidence-based protocols provides motivation for continued improvement.
- Improved compliance with sepsis protocols can reduce sepsis mortality across a health care system.

INTRODUCTION

Since the early 2000s, much effort has gone into reducing morbidity and mortality associated with severe sepsis and septic shock. In 2001, Rivers and colleagues[1] published the sentinel article on early goal-directed therapy in treating severe sepsis and septic shock. In 2002, the Surviving Sepsis Campaign was introduced to raise awareness and improve care of patients with sepsis.[2] In 2004, the *Journal of Critical Care Medicine* published the Surviving Sepsis Guidelines for Management of Severe Sepsis and Septic Shock to improve care and outcomes of critically ill patients with

Disclosures: The authors have nothing to disclose.
[a] Office of the Chief Nursing Officer, Baylor Scott & White–North Texas, 2001 Bryan Street, Suite 600, Dallas, TX 75201, USA; [b] Department of Critical Care, Baylor University Medical Center at Dallas, 3500 Gaston Avenue, Dallas, TX 75246, USA
* Corresponding author.
E-mail address: KrisP@baylorhealth.edu

Crit Care Nurs Clin N Am 26 (2014) 487–498
http://dx.doi.org/10.1016/j.ccell.2014.08.005
0899-5885/14/$ – see front matter © 2014 Elsevier Inc. All rights reserved.

sepsis.[3] In response to these evidence-based guidelines, hospitals and health care providers began implementing recommended sepsis care bundles to improve recognition, treatment, and outcomes of severe sepsis and septic shock. Despite these efforts, hospital death rates for septicemia as a primary diagnosis increased 17% between 2000 and 2010 (13.9 deaths per 100 admissions in 2000 compared with 16.3 deaths per 100 admissions in 2010), whereas overall hospital death rates have decreased.[4] For patients with severe sepsis, the mortality rate is still almost one out of every three patients.[5] In 2010, sepsis was recognized as the 11th leading cause of death in the United States[6] and was one of the top 10 leading causes of death in the younger age groups from birth to 14 years and the age group of 55 years or older.[7] Septicemia also has severe economic consequences and was identified as the most expensive condition to treat in US hospitals, accounting for 5.2% of total aggregate costs.[8]

SEPSIS AND HEALTH CARE: A SYSTEMS VIEW
Sepsis and the Human Body: A Systems View

Sepsis is recognized as a complicated and dynamic disease state involving multiple processes and physiologic responses within the human body.[9] Understanding and predicting the pathophysiology of sepsis in any one patient is difficult because the human body is also a complex adaptive system.[10] At the Merinoff Symposium on Sepsis in Fall 2010, a group of international stakeholders developed consensus on public and molecular definitions of sepsis as "a life threatening condition that arises when the body's response to an infection injures its own tissues and organs," which occurs as a result of "unbalanced activation of innate immunity."[11] This definition provides a more accurate description of sepsis as a complex disease syndrome that occurs within the complex processes of the human body.

Performance Improvement in a Complex Adaptive System

Baylor Health Care System (BHCS) is a large health care system of multiple facilities, departments, services, and staff, all with multiple and important priorities in the areas of quality, service, people, and finance. Reducing sepsis mortality across this complex health care system requires a systems approach to performance improvement (PI). Tsasis and coworkers[12] report that change in integrated care processes is difficult in health care systems because of a lack of understanding of complex adaptive systems and suggest that "health systems integration requires policies and management practices that support relationship building and information-sharing across organizational and professional boundaries, and that recognize change as an evolving learning process rather than a series of programmatic steps."

Kottke and coworkers[13] identified five rules that can create value in health care systems: (1) identification of measurable goals that are aligned among stakeholders, (2) transparency in public reporting, (3) adequate and available resources, (4) alignment of incentives with goals, and (5) engaged leadership. Funk and coworkers[14] described the need for a multidisciplinary approach to improving sepsis care, which calls for active involvement of executive leadership and direct caregivers within a program of continuous assessment and reporting of outcomes. In *Achieving STEEEP Health Care*, Luquire[15] cites the importance of strong nursing leadership, a shared governance model, and standardization of care to best practices. In the journey to drive a reduction in sepsis mortality, the BHCS has demonstrated a robust systems approach to PI following the principles outlined in **Box 1** and by deploying a variety of strategies and tactics.

> **Box 1**
> **Performance improvement principles in health care systems**
>
> 1. Setting of measurable goals with alignment among stakeholders[13]
> 2. Transparency in public reporting[13]
> 3. Adequate and available resources[13]
> 4. Alignment of incentives with goals[13]
> 5. Engaged leadership[13]/executive and direct care provider involvement[14]
> 6. Multidisciplinary approach[14]
> 7. Continuous quality improvement approach with emphasis on targeted outcomes[14]
> 8. Strong nursing leadership[15]
> 9. Shared governance model[15]
> 10. Standardization of care to best practices[15]
>
> *Data from* Refs.[13–15]

STRATEGIES AND TACTICS TO IMPROVE SEPSIS CARE AND REDUCE MORTALITY
Goal Setting

Goal setting for sepsis care and outcomes occurs at the health care system executive level and is cascaded to hospital executives, nurse and physician leadership, service line councils, emergency department (ED) and critical care unit leaders, and direct care providers. This method of cascading goals results in alignment of efforts and re-sources throughout the organization. Goals must outline specific targets and time-frames and must be measurable.

The BHCS ED council developed compliance goals for the ED service line that included specific targets for a 3-hour care bundle in a selected group of high-risk patients with a positive sepsis screen at triage. A standard was set for routine sepsis screening of all ED patients greater than 16 years old and a routine screening process was implemented across all system EDs. The group identified goals (**Box 2**) for patients who screen positive or who are admitted with a diagnosis of severe sepsis or septic shock and a standard monthly report was formatted for sharing with hospital staff and leadership.

Transparency in Reporting

Rigorous and objective chart audits, data collection, and reporting are coordinated through the BHCS Office of Patient Safety. Care process and mortality reports are shared with personnel at all levels of the organization from direct caregivers to board

> **Box 2**
> **BHCS ED council goals for care processes in patients with severe sepsis and septic shock**
>
> • Triage time to lactate: mean time less than 180 minutes
> • Triage time to completion of intravenous fluid bolus of 30 mL/kg: mean time less than 180 minutes
> • Triage time to administration of appropriate antibiotics: mean time less than 180 minutes
> • Triage to transfer to definitive care unit: mean time less than 180 minutes

members. Unblinded hospital data and aggregate reports are reviewed and discussed at system and hospital board meetings, best care committees, mortality review meetings, sepsis care steering teams, ED and critical care service line councils, unit-based practice councils, and departmental staff meetings.

A key initiative in fiscal year 2013 was the implementation of daily staff huddles on sepsis care in the ED. All EDs implemented huddle boards with daily updates that include the number of patients with a positive sepsis screen and compliance with antibiotic administration and intravenous (IV) fluid bolus completion within 180 minutes. The daily huddles occur face-to-face with oncoming staff at change of shift. The daily shift huddles provide a venue for reward and recognition following high-compliance days and for discussion of improvement strategies when compliance is low.

At Baylor University Medical Center, the rapid response team (RRT) reports all transfer delays directly to the vice president of critical care. The details of the delay are routed to the chief medical officer if physician-related, the nurse manager if nurse-related, or the administrative supervisor if related to bed availability. A drill down review occurs to discuss process improvement strategies. The process has resulted in implementation of a "bed ahead" concept where a patient room is always cleared anticipating the next sepsis patient admission and has demonstrated a marked reduction in transfer times to the intensive care unit (ICU).

Resource Availability

To meet best care standards for patients with severe sepsis and septic shock, multiple resources were developed and/or allocated for clinical and reporting processes.

- Education programs developed and placed on the Baylor Learning Network online education application
- Administrative support received for key clinical leaders to attend national conferences and symposiums on sepsis care
- Sepsis screening tool (paper and electronic) developed for ED triage nurses
- Code sepsis algorithm developed to expedite needed resources to the patient bedside and guide care to established evidence-based practice standards
- Difficult IV protocol developed to expedite IV fluid bolus
- RRT protocol developed for response to the ED to provide assistance and facilitate admission
- Appropriate antibiotics stocked in unit medication dispensing systems in the ED and ICUs
- The RRT order sets revised to include sepsis screening
- Sepsis care tracking and reporting tools developed
- ED information system programmed to place a color-coded marker to highlight patients with positive sepsis screen
- Office of Patient Safety developed job position for registered nurse sepsis chart auditor
- Resuscitation and admission order sets developed for sepsis

Alignment of Incentives with Goals

Achievement of sepsis care performance goals is tied to the annual performance appraisal process and financial merit increases for clinical staff and hospital leadership. The emergency physicians group has implemented sepsis care goals for individual physicians and has linked financial incentives to the goals. By aligning incentives with goals, individuals at all levels are motivated to prioritize the actions needed to meet specified targets.

Engaged Leadership/Executive and Direct Caregiver Involvement

To achieve sepsis goals and improved patient outcomes, all levels of staff are expected to engage and support PI initiatives in a manner congruent with their role. Engagement and involvement are encouraged through the setting of specific goals and aligning incentives with those goals. The impetus for ongoing improvement stems from the BHCS vision "to be trusted as the best place to give and receive safe, quality, compassionate care."[16] High levels of staff support result in a more engaged workforce that aligns with system priorities in the delivery of safe, timely, effective, efficient, equitable, patient-centered (STEEEP) care (**Box 3**).

Engaged leadership at BHCS creates a high-performing culture and ensures appropriate resources to assist direct care staff with achieving goals. System and hospital leadership sit at the same table as direct caregivers to track progress toward goals and develop strategies for ongoing improvement in sepsis care. Active involvement of leadership and direct care staff occurs in quality meetings at every level including system and hospital board meetings, quality meetings, service line councils, and unit-based practice councils.

Multidisciplinary Approach

Severe sepsis and septic shock are complex conditions that warrant a rapid response and multidisciplinary approach. Clinical resources that are necessary in the management of care include ED nurses, physicians, and support staff; access services; laboratory services; radiology and imaging services; pharmacy; hospitalists; intensive care nurses; critical care and consulting physicians; and cardiopulmonary services. Additional support services may include nutrition, social work, care coordination, physical medicine and rehabilitation services, pastoral care, supply chain management, medical records, nurse educators, and discharge planners.

PI planning includes representation from the clinical services listed previously and health care improvement, Office of Patient Safety, decision support services, performance measurement and reporting, LEAN operations, information systems, advanced practice nurses, executive leadership, nursing and physician leaders, and direct care clinicians.

Continuous Quality Improvement Approach to Performance Improvement

The BHCS STEEEP Academy was developed to provide training for hospital leaders on continuous quality improvement principles and methods.[17] Participants in the STEEEP Academy apply new knowledge and tools in a selected PI project. Successful

---

Box 3
STEEEP health care

- Safe
- Timely
- Effective
- Efficient
- Equitable
- Patient-centered

From Leonard BM, Shutts C, Fleming NS. STEEEP Academy. In: Ballard D, editor. Achieving STEEEP health care. Boca Raton (FL): CRC Press; 2013. p. 53–63.

initiatives are recognized and shared across the health care system to spread best practices.

Sepsis PI projects using STEEEP Academy principles have resulted in improved care for patients with sepsis. Using a Plan-Do-Check-Act approach, Baylor University Medical Center reduced time from ED to ICU admission for patients with severe sepsis from 507 minutes (8.5 hours) in June 2011 to 281 minutes (4.7 hours) in June 2012, an improvement of almost 4 hours (**Box 4, Fig. 1**).

Strong Nursing Leadership

The role of nursing leadership in driving quality initiatives in sepsis care cannot be understated. Nursing leaders at BHCS are actively engaged in planning and implementing PI initiatives that have resulted in better care and outcomes for patients with sepsis. Nurse leaders cochair the emergency and critical care service line councils with physician champions. These councils partner with other physician leaders, nurse leaders, and other support services across the health care system. Nurses also take active leadership roles in sepsis care steering teams at the system level and at the

---

Box 4
Plan-Do-Check-Act approach to reducing ED to ICU times for severe sepsis admissions at Baylor University Medical Center

PLAN: In 2011, ED to ICU admission times at Baylor University Medical Center averaged between 7.0 and 8.5 hours for patients with severe sepsis. A multidisciplinary team led by the vice president of critical care services and director of emergency services met and developed plans to improve the process and hold accountability for expediting ICU care of patients with severe sepsis and septic shock.

DO: Multiple activities were implemented and are outlined next:

- The RRT, administrative nursing supervisor, ED nursing supervisor, and room control were immediately notified by the ED when a code sepsis was activated.

- The ED physician would consult directly with the admitting physician to expedite admission orders.

- The RRT nurse responded to the ED for code sepsis patients and worked with the admitting medical doctor to get the sepsis admission order set signed.

- The RRT nurse would coordinate the transfer with the ICU and transport team. ICU staff would assist the transport team and ED nurse as needed to transport the patient to the ICU. A patient report handoff would occur directly with the ED registered nurse caring for the patient to the ICU registered nurse caring for the patient.

- The vice president of critical care services began carrying the RRT pager and would call the RRT nurse to follow up on every sepsis RRT page. The intent was to assist the RRT and ED nurses with eliminating obstacles to ICU admission.

- A "bed ahead" protocol was implemented so that an ICU bed would always be available for a sepsis patient admission.

- Weekly sepsis review meetings were scheduled with the vice president of critical care services, RRT manager, ED manager, and an ED staff nurse to review ICU sepsis admissions from the previous week and discuss issues and solutions.

CHECK: The time frame for ED to ICU admission at Baylor University Medical Center was reduced from 507 minutes (8.5 hours) in June 2011 to 280 minutes (4.7 hours) in June 2012, an improvement of almost 4 hours.

ACT: ED and ICU staff acquired a higher level of awareness and a sense of urgency to move patients with severe sepsis from the ED to ICU and processes were hardwired. The results have been sustained and the average for July to October 2013 remains less than 300 minutes.

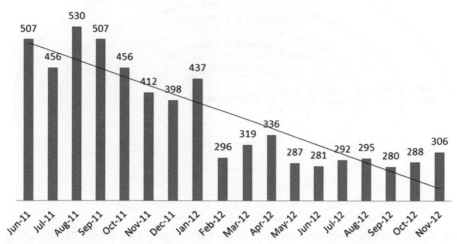

ED Arrival to ICU (min)

Fig. 1. The time frame for ED to ICU admission at Baylor University Medical Center was reduced from 507 minutes (8.5 hours) in June 2011 to 280 minutes (4.7 hours) in June 2012, an improvement of almost 4 hours.

individual hospitals. The BHCS senior vice president and chief nursing officer is the executive sponsor of the emergency and critical care councils.

Nurse leaders attend the STEEEP Academy training and take on leadership roles in planning and implementing PI initiatives. Nurse-driven processes in sepsis screening, initiation of diagnostic protocols to measure lactate levels, and daily staff huddles have resulted in significant improvements in antibiotic and IV fluid bolus administration for the sepsis patient population in the ED setting.

Shared Governance Model

A robust shared governance model serves to promote authority, autonomy, and accountability in professional nursing practice at all levels in the organization.[18] The BHCS shared governance structure (**Fig. 2**) represents the structure of nurse decision-making with the patient at the center of care and the bedside nurse being supported by unit, facility, and system councils. Sepsis improvement initiatives and performance reports are discussed at all levels of shared governance.

Standardization to Evidence-Based and Best Care Practices

The Institute of Medicine emphasized the importance of evidence-based practice in the 2001 publication *Crossing the Quality Chasm: A New Health System for the 21st Century*.[19] The BHCS developed sepsis screening tools and order sets in 2009 based on Surviving Sepsis Campaign guidelines and published updates[3,20,21] and Institute for Healthcare Improvement resources.[22] The Sepsis Screening Form and Sepsis Resuscitation and Admission Order sets have since been converted to tools in the electronic health record in the ED and inpatient settings.

RESULTS
Process Improvements in Clinical Care

The BHCS began measuring and reporting key metrics in sepsis care in 2010. The reports included median times by facility for key processes including ED arrival to lactate

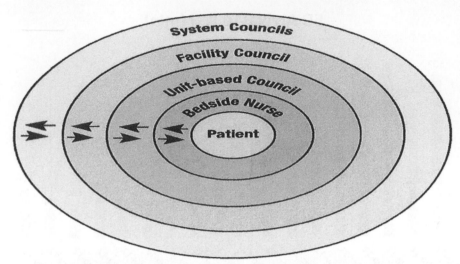

Fig. 2. BHCS shared governance structure. (*From* Baylor Health Care System. Baylor nursing [July 2010 – Jun 2011] annual report. Dallas (TX): Baylor Health Care System; 2011; with permission.)

testing, antibiotic administration, IV fluid bolus, and transition time to the ICU. The BHCS emergency department council used these data to help drive improvements through sharing of best practices and friendly competition. In 2011, the reports were updated to include aggregate data for the system and additional measures to evaluate compliance with individual and bundled sepsis care goals. Although average times were well within the 180-minute goal, adding a compliance measure of 80% motivated clinicians to improve care for a larger percentage of patients. The following results were observed:

- BHCS median time from ED arrival to antibiotic administration dropped from 122 minutes to 74 minutes (**Fig. 3**)
- BHCS median time from ED arrival to completion of IV fluid bolus dropped from 119 minutes to 88 minutes (**Fig. 4**)
- BHCS compliance for time of ED arrival to antibiotic administration within 180 minutes improved from 70% to 90% (**Fig. 5**)

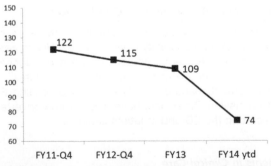

Fig. 3. Baylor Health Care System median time from emergency department arrival to antibiotic administration decreased from 122 minutes to 74 minutes. FY, fiscal year; ytd, year to date.

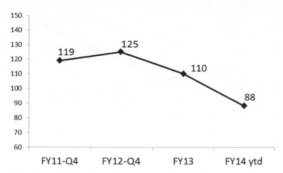

Fig. 4. Baylor Health Care System median time from emergency department arrival to completion of intravenous fluid bolus decreased from 119 minutes to 88 minutes. FY, fiscal year; ytd, year to date.

- BHCS compliance for time of ED arrival to completion of IV fluid bolus within 180 minutes improved from 56% to 83% (**Fig. 6**)

Reduction in Sepsis Mortality

BHCS also tracks and reports sepsis mortality. The hospital standard mortality ratio (HSMR) metric is used to report the ratio of actual deaths to expected deaths multiplied by 100. When the count of actual deaths exceeds the count of expected deaths the HSMR is greater than 100. From fiscal year 2007 to fiscal year 2013, the BHCS reduced sepsis mortality measures as HSMR from 120.5 to 75.4 (**Fig. 7**). The variance in actual versus expected deaths is also tracked and reported as patient lives saved or lost. From fiscal year 2009 to fiscal year 2013, 555 patient lives were saved as a result of improved sepsis care processes and reduced mortality (**Fig. 8**).

ONGOING CHALLENGES AND NEXT STEPS

BHCS maintains a culture of continuous quality improvement. Efforts persist to improve processes and available resources in delivery of sepsis care. The following activities are planned or are currently in progress to support ongoing improvement efforts:

- Complete implementation of the electronic health record in all BHCS facilities.
- Optimize workflows between the ED and inpatient units for sepsis admissions by leveraging improvements in technology and the electronic health record.

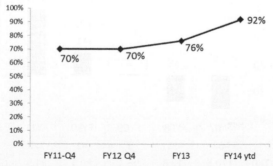

Fig. 5. Baylor Health Care System compliance for time of emergency department arrival to antibiotic administration within 180 minutes improved from 70% to 90%. FY, fiscal year; ytd, year to date.

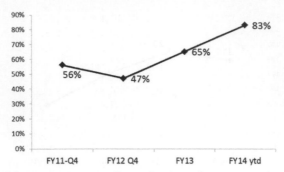

Fig. 6. Baylor Health Care System compliance for time of emergency department arrival to completion of intravenous fluid bolus within 180 minutes improved from 56% to 83%. FY, fiscal year; ytd, year to date.

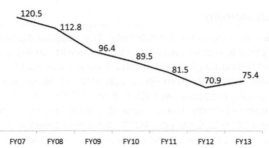

Fig. 7. Baylor Health Care System demonstrated a reduction in sepsis mortality (HSMR) from 120.5 to 75.4. FY, fiscal year.

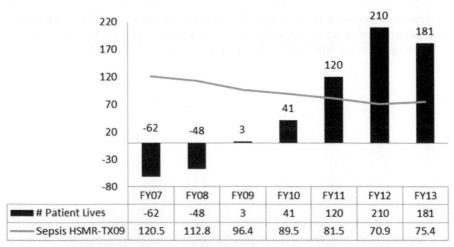

	FY07	FY08	FY09	FY10	FY11	FY12	FY13
■ # Patient Lives	-62	-48	3	41	120	210	181
— Sepsis HSMR-TX09	120.5	112.8	96.4	89.5	81.5	70.9	75.4

Fig. 8. From FY09 to FY13, 555 patient lives have been saved at Baylor Health Care System as a result of improved sepsis care processes and reduction in mortality. FY, fiscal year.

- Implement routine sepsis screening for inpatients.
- Measure and report inpatient metrics for sepsis care.
- Measure and report compliance with the updated 2012 Surviving Sepsis Campaign 6-hour care bundle, which includes use of vasopressors for persistent hypotension after fluid resuscitation, measurement of central venous pressure and central venous oxygen saturation if initial lactate level greater than or equal to 4 mmol/dL or persistent hypotension after fluid resuscitation, and repeat lactate testing when initial lactate is elevated.[21]
- Update sepsis resuscitation and admission order sets according to the 2012 Surviving Sepsis Campaign revisions.
- Partner with prehospital care providers to facilitate initiation of routine sepsis screening, diagnostics, and treatment before ED arrival.
- Develop and provide sepsis awareness education in the community.
- Share successes and lessons learned internally and externally.

SUMMARY

A strong and consistent focus on sepsis care in the BHCS has resulted in improved processes and reduced sepsis mortality across the health care system. An organized approach to continuous quality improvement, support and engagement of executive leadership, nursing and physician leaders, and direct care staff, and rigorous goal setting and tracking of metrics with transparent reporting are strategies that have been the most impactful in this large complex health care system.

REFERENCES

1. Rivers E, Nguyen B, Havsted S, et al. Early goal-directed therapy in the treatment of severe sepsis and septic shock. N Engl J Med 2001;345(19):1368–77.
2. Surviving Sepsis Campaign History. Surviving Sepsis Campaign Web site. Available at: http://www.survivingsepsis.org/AboutSSC/Pages/History.aspx. Accessed November 22, 2013.
3. Dellinger RP, Carlet JM, Masur H, et al. Surviving sepsis campaign guide. Crit Care Med 2004;32(3):858–73. Available at: http://www.esicm.org/upload/SSCGuidelines%20ICM%20March%2004.pdf. Accessed November 22, 2013.
4. Hall MJ, Levant S, DeFrances CJ. Trends in inpatient hospital deaths: National Hospital Discharge Survey, 2000–2010. Hyattsville (MD): National Center for Health Statistics; 2013. NCHS data brief, no 118. Available at: http://www.cdc.gov/nchs/data/databriefs/db118.htm. Accessed November 22, 2013.
5. Stevenson EK, Rubenstein AR, Radin GT, et al. Two decades of mortality trends among patients with severe sepsis: a comparative meta-analysis. Crit Care Med 2014;42:1–7. http://dx.doi.org/10.1097/CCM.0000000000000026.
6. Murphy S, Xu J, Kochanek KD. Deaths: final data for 2010. Natl Vital Stat Rep 2013;61(4). Available at: http://www.cdc.gov/nchs/data/nvsr/nvsr61/nvsr61-04.pdf. Accessed November 30, 2013. p. 1.
7. 10 Leading Causes of Death by Age Group, United States–2010. National Center for Injury Prevention and Control Web site. Available at: http://www.cdc.gov/injury/wisqars/pdf/10LCIDAllDeathsByAgeGroup2010-a.pdf. Accessed November 30, 2013.
8. Torio CM, Andrews RM. National inpatient hospital costs: the most expensive conditions by payer. Rockville (MD): Agency for Healthcare Research and Quality; 2013. HCUP Statistical Brief #160. Available at: http://www.hcupus.ahrq.gov/reports/statbriefs/sb160.pdf. Accessed November 30, 2013.

9. Namas R, Zamora R, Namas R, et al. Sepsis: something old, something new, and a systems view. J Crit Care 2012;27(3):314.e1–11. Available at: http://www.ncbi.nlm.nih.gov/pmc/articles/PMC3206132/. Accessed November 30, 2013.

10. Mann-Salinas LE, Engebretson J, Batchinsky A. A complex systems view of sepsis: implications for nursing. Dimens Crit Care Nurs 2013;32(1):12–7. http://dx.doi.org/10.1097/DCC.0b013e31827680e4. Available at OvidSP with full text. Accessed November 30, 2013.

11. Czura CJ. Merinoff Symposium 2010: sepsis—speaking with one voice. Mol Med 2011;17(1–2):2–3. Available at: http://www.ncbi.nlm.nih.gov/pmc/articles/PMC30 22986/. Accessed November 30, 2013.

12. Tsasis P, Evans JM, Owen S. Reframing the challenges to integrated care: a complex-adaptive systems perspective. Int J Integrated Care 2012;12. NBN: NL: UI:10-1-113786. Available at: http://www.ijic.org/index.php/ijic/article/view/URN. Accessed November 25, 2013.

13. Kottke TE, Pronk NP, Isham GJ. The simple health system rules that create value. Prev Chronic Dis 2012;9:110179. Available at: http://www.ncbi.nlm.nih.gov/pmc/articles/PMC3340212/. Accessed November 25, 2013.

14. Funk D, Sebat F, Kumar A. A systems approach to the early recognition and rapid administration of best practice therapy in sepsis and septic shock. Curr Opin Crit Care 2009;15(4):301–7. Available at: OvidSP with full text. Accessed November 22, 2013.

15. Luquire R. Nursing leadership (chapter 7). In: Ballard D, editor. Achieving STEEEP health care. Boca Raton (FL): CRC Press; 2013. p. 43–50.

16. Mission, Vision, and Values. Baylor Health Care System Web site. 2013. Available at: https://www.mybaylor.com/Aboutus/Mission/Pages/default.aspx. Accessed December 10, 2013.

17. Leonard BM, Shutts C, Fleming NS. STEEEP academy (chapter 8). In: Ballard D, editor. Achieving STEEEP health care. Boca Raton (FL): CRC Press; 2013. p. 53–63.

18. Baylor nursing annual report: July 2010 through June 2011. Dallas (TX): Baylor Health Care System; 2012.

19. Crossing the quality chasm: a new health system for the 21st century – executive summary. Institute of Medicine Committee on Quality of Health Care in America; 2001. Available at: http://www.ahrmm.org/ahrmm/newsandissues/issuesandini tiatives/IOM6/files/IOM.pdf. Accessed December 12, 2013.

20. Dellinger RP, Levy MM, Carlet JM, et al. Surviving Sepsis Campaign: international guidelines for management of severe sepsis and septic shock: 2008. Intensive Care Med 2008;34:17–60. Available at: http://www.ncbi.nlm.nih.gov/pmc/articles/PMC2249616/pdf/134_2007_Article_934.pdf. Accessed December 15, 2013.

21. Dellinger RP, Levy MM, Rhodes A, et al. Surviving Sepsis Campaign: international guidelines for management of severe sepsis and septic shock: 2012. Crit Care Med 2013;41(2):580–637. Available at: http://www.sccm.org/Documents/SSC-Guidelines.pdf. Accessed November 22, 2013.

22. Evaluation for Severe Sepsis Screening Tool. Surviving Sepsis Campaign and Institute for Healthcare Improvement. 2005. Available at: http://www.ihi.org/IHI/Topics/CriticalCare/Sepsis. Accessed December 5, 2009.

Implications and Interventions Related to Obstructive Sleep Apnea

Amy Veenstra, RN, CCRN, CMC[a],*,
Emylene Untalan, MSN, RN, CCRN, CPAN[b]

KEYWORDS

- Obstructive sleep apnea • Hypopnea • Complications • Risk factors
- STOP-Bang questionnaire

KEY POINTS

- Obstructive sleep apnea (OSA) patients are at increased risk for postoperative complications.
- A high percentage of surgical patients with OSA are undiagnosed.
- Validated screening helps identify patients at high risk for OSA.
- Identification, treatment, and monitoring can decrease complications.

Obstructive sleep apnea (OSA) contributes to the risk of postoperative complications of individuals undergoing surgery. Patients with OSA are at higher risk for many different negative outcomes such as hypercapnia, oxygen desaturation, reintubation, cardiac arrhythmias, cardiac arrest, delirium, transfer to the ICU, increased length of stay in the hospital, and death.[1–4] The overall complication rate for OSA subjects undergoing surgery is 44% compared with 28% of those without OSA. The highest complication rates are related to respiratory issues.[1] In a study by Gupta and colleagues, OSA subjects undergoing hip or knee replacement had serious complications of 24% as compared to 9% in the non-OSA group.[3] The overall complication rate in the OSA group was 39% and 18% in the control group. A study of orthopedic and general surgery subjects found the OSA subjects in both groups had higher postoperative rates of aspiration, adult respiratory distress syndrome, and intubation or mechanical ventilation.[5]

Disclosures: None applicable.
[a] Nursing Administration, Baylor University Medical Center at Dallas, 3500 Gaston Avenue, Dallas, TX 75246, USA; [b] Post Anesthesia Care Unit, Baylor University Medical Center at Dallas, 3500 Gaston Avenue, Dallas, TX 75246, USA
* Corresponding author.
E-mail address: amyv@baylorhealth.edu

Crit Care Nurs Clin N Am 26 (2014) 499–509
http://dx.doi.org/10.1016/j.ccell.2014.08.015
0899-5885/14/$ – see front matter © 2014 Elsevier Inc. All rights reserved.

Our hospital is not immune from the negative impact that OSA can have on surgical patients. A patient under went an elective orthopedic surgery was found unresponsive postoperatively. CPR was performed but the patient expired within 24 hours of surgery. The patient had a history of sleep apnea and obesity, was on patient-controlled analgesia (PCA), and was found with the head of the bed flat. Another patient died postoperatively after being found unresponsive, despite resuscitative measures. This patient also had a history of sleep apnea and was on PCA but had a low body mass index (BMI).

A multidisciplinary group was formed to examine patient factors that contribute to a high risk for postoperative respiratory depression such as underlying comorbidities, suspected or diagnosed sleep apnea, and intolerance of opioids. The committee also reviewed processes and procedures that might lead or contribute to adverse postoperative events, as well as ensure that evidence-based practices are being used when caring for patients having surgery.

The purpose of this article is to describe our findings and actions related to preventing OSA related deaths.

DEFINITION

Hypopnea is a respiratory event that is abnormal, resulting in at least 30% reduction of airflow compared with baseline, 4% or greater oxygen desaturation, both lasting at least 10 seconds.[6] Hypopnea can also be a 50% or less reduction in airflow lasting for 10 seconds, with a drop in oxygen saturation of less than 3% or an arousal from sleep.[6,7] Apnea is clinically defined as the absence of airflow for at least 10 seconds with continued ventilatory effort even though the flow of air has ceased.[6,7] The research definition of apnea is similar to that of hypopnea but includes the decrease of oxygen saturation sustained for at least 10 seconds.[6,7] In central apnea airflow halts for at least 10 seconds and there is no effort to take a breath. Mixed apnea begins as central apnea but toward the end there is a ventilatory effort but no airflow, with the event lasting for at least 10 seconds.[6,7]

American Academy of Sleep Medicine (AASM) developed criteria that looks at polysomnography (PSG) results and observed or reported symptoms to help diagnose OSA. PSG is recommended for identifying individuals with OSA. Monitoring equipment includes an electroencephalogram to assess stages of sleep, an electromyogram to measure muscle activity in the chin and legs, and an electrocardiogram (ECG) to monitor for cardiac arrhythmias.[7] Apnea is measured with an oronasal thermal sensor and pulse oximetry is also monitored.[7] The results of the PSG quantify the number of apnea and hypopnea events reported as an apnea-hypopnea index (AHI). The AHI helps classify OSA as mild, moderate, or severe, as defined by AASM (Table 1).[8]

Table 1 Classification of OSA	
Classification	API
Mild	5–15 apnea or hypopnea events per hour
Moderate	15–30 apnea or hypopnea events per hour
Severe	>30 apnea or hypopnea events per hour and/or hypoxia <90% for >20% of total sleep time

Adapted from Gutierrez C, Brady P. Obstructive sleep apnea: a diagnostic and treatment guide. J Fam Pract 2013;62(10):570.

PATHOPHYSIOLOGY

Collapse of the airway can occur behind the soft palate, from the soft palate to the epiglottis, and/or from the epiglottis to the larynx, leading to decreased and turbulent airflow or obstruction.[9,10] Anatomic abnormalities such as displacement of the hyoid bone, shortening or hypoplasia of the mandible and maxilla, and a longer pharynx, contribute to the development of OSA.[9,10] Enlargement of soft tissues such as the tongue, soft palate, tonsils, lymphatic tissue, pharyngeal fat pads, pharyngeal mucosa, and upper airway (UA) muscles can decrease the patency of the airway due to inflammation, swelling, and hypertrophy.[9,10] The pharyngeal muscles are required for many different tasks of the UA, including respiration, coughing, and movement of the tongue and pharynx. The pharyngeal dilator muscles play a crucial role in maintaining patency of the UA.[10] The UA dilator muscles are controlled through many different physiologic means and variation may contribute to the development of OSA.

The central respiratory pattern-generating neurons located in the ventral medulla stimulate the UA dilating muscles just before the diaphragm contracts. This ensures that the UA dilating muscles are able to overcome the negative pressure during inspiration, maintaining airway patency.[9] The central respiratory pattern-generating neurons also respond to changes in Po_2 and Pco_2.[10] There is a risk of OSA occurring if the neural drive to the diaphragm and the dilating muscles of the UA are not sufficient or are not coordinated with each other.[11]

The negative intrapharyngeal pressure also prompts a response from the pharyngeal muscles to ensure the airway is open.[9,10] Deterioration of this reflex may be caused by trauma and inflammation due to snoring vibration and repetitious collapse of the UA.[9,10,12] The state sensitive neural systems have heightened activity during wakefulness but during sleep the normal response of the pharyngeal dilator muscles to protect the patency of the airway fails as the muscles relax and pharyngeal collapse occurs.[9,10]

Sleep has a significant effect on the different pharyngeal muscles. Some of the muscles recover to waking activity shortly after sleep occurs, whereas other UA muscles continue to lose activity as sleep deepens, as much as 70% to 80%, causing an increase in UA resistance.[9] During sleep, lung volumes are decreased. Increased lung volume contributes to the size of the UA and contributes to caudal traction, increasing the stiffness of the airway, decreasing the risk for collapse.[9-11] Rapid eye movement (REM) sleep contributes to more events of partial or complete obstruction because the UA muscle activation and negative intrapharyngeal pressure response are more depressed during REM than in the other stages of sleep.[13]

PREVALENCE AND RISK FACTORS

Studies have shown that one of every five adults has at least mild OSA and one of every 15 adults has at least moderate OSA.[14] There is a concern that as many as 75% to 80% of OSA cases are undiagnosed, leaving at-risk individuals untreated.[15] Undiagnosed sleep-disordered breathing with an AHI less than five occurrence rate is 9% in women and 24% rate in men.[16] It is not clear why there is a two to threefold increase in the risk for men compared with women. Chronic diseases, health behaviors, environmental, and occupational exposures may be contributing factors.[14] Another factor might be the protective effects of hormones found in premenopausal women. Progesterone may contribute to respiratory control system and testosterone contributes to development of pharyngeal fat.[10] Different studies show that postmenopausal women are more at risk for OSA than premenopausal women. Hormone replacement therapy users have half the risk of those not on replacement therapy.[14,15]

Ethnicity is considered a risk factor with African Americans at a higher risk than whites.[17] Although only African American men were at a greater risk than white men there is no difference in the risk between the women.[14] Asians also have a higher rate of OSA than whites and it is more severe.[10,15]

The prevalence of OSA increases with age. There is a marked increase in the rates of OSA in the middle-aged compared with the elderly.[14] This twofold to threefold increase plateaus after 65 years of age.[15] With age, the reflex reaction of the UA muscles to the negative pressure in the pharynx deteriorates. There are greater deposits of fat around the pharynx even though weight management is not a concern.[18] Studies have shown a familial link, so genetics may predispose individuals to the development of OSA.[15,18] Anatomy, traits, respiratory responses, and ventilatory control may be genetically linked.[18]

Smoking causes inflammation in the airways and sleep instability (due to decreased nicotine levels), placing the patient at risk for OSA.[14,15] Alcohol, craniofacial abnormalities (posttrauma, surgery, or congenital), and nasal congestion (infection, allergies) place patients at risk for developing OSA.[10,14,15] Many studies have shown that obesity is the largest risk factor for OSA.[14] A pattern of fat disposition in the abdomen, upper body, and neck has a higher incidence than fat disposition to the hips and thighs.[10,14,15] At least 40% of those suffering from obesity have OSA and 70% of individuals with OSA are obese (BMI $\geq$30 kg/m^2).[8] The physiologic effects include reduction in lung volumes and functional residual capacity due to abdominal fat. Pharyngeal fat leads to a narrowing of the airway, increasing the risk of collapse.[18] There is a sixfold increased chance of developing moderate or severe OSA for those with a 10% weight gain.[14] Many other studies show a reduction in AHI with weight reduction.[14,15]

SURGICAL RISK

Finkel, and colleagues, found that 23.7% of surgical subjects screened as high risk for OSA yet 80.7% of those subjects were undiagnosed.[19] The surgical OSA patient is at higher risk of complications in the perioperative period due to the effects of sedation, anesthesia, and the use of opioids.[19] The negative intrapharyngeal pressure reflex is compromised. Less of this protective reflex can lead to an increase in apneic events, as well as in the length of apnea, and there is depression of the central respiratory output to the UA muscles.[19,20]

Anesthetics, sedation, and analgesia affect the control of breathing in varying ways such as chemoreceptor depression, loss of tonic activity, and inhibition of muscle activity.[20] The respiratory system is less responsive to hypercapnia and hypoxemia.[21] Surgery disrupts REM sleep the first night after surgery due to the increase in catecholamine and cortisol levels.[22] REM rebound occurs when REM sleep returns (second or third night, although it may occur later). There is an increased duration and density causing a threefold increase in hypoxemic events.[21,22] Surgical patients are often placed in the supine position due to the procedure. Postoperatively they do not want to move due to pain, intravenous lines, and other invasive tubes. The supine position contributes to obstructive events for patients with OSA. At least 60% of patients with OSA sleep predominantly in the supine position.[23] Functional residual capacity and expiratory reserve capacity decrease from the upright or lateral position to the supine position.[23] These changes occurred dramatically in obese individuals with BMIs greater than 25 to 30 kg/m^2.[23] REM rebound, pharmacologic agents, and the supine position could act together to aggravate or worsen OSA.[21,24]

Depression of the respiratory response mechanisms and UA muscle relaxation places the postoperative patient at risk for aspiration and pneumonia.[5] Surgical patients have sympathetic activation due to the surgical stress and hypoxemic events during REM sleep. This increase of sympathetic activation can profoundly lead to an increase in mean arterial pressure and hemodynamic instability, including ischemia and infarction.[21,25] Large blood pressure changes occur from obstruction and response to vasopressors is compromised with the chronic adrenergic response.[21] Delirium can occur from lack of REM sleep, which can lead to irritability, impaired memory, and impaired learning.[21] Sleep deprivation can also lead to impaired respiratory response to hypoxia and hypercapnia.[21] Cardiac arrhythmias occur due to hypoxemia with the development of atrial fibrillation having a 4.5 odds ratio compared with control subjects.[21]

IMPLEMENTATION OF STRATEGIES FOR DECREASING POSTOPERATIVE COMPLICATIONS

The multidisciplinary team consisted of physicians (anesthesia, pulmonary, patient safety), pharmacists, registered nurses (orthopedics, patient safety, postanesthesia care unit [PACU], rapid response team [RRT], risk management, respiratory care, and administration. The Post Operative Respiratory Depression Committee reviewed RRT oversedation events, these identified that orthopedics patients who failed their oxygen withdrawal trial in the PACU have the greatest risk for an oversedation event. Three key factors for adverse events are equal or greater than 60 years of age, BMI equal to or greater than 30 kg/m^2, and intolerance of opioids.

A Respiratory Arrest Risk Alert was created by the committee to assist the medical staff to identify patients who are at high risk for postoperative respiratory depression. This includes patients on PCA and known or suspected OSA. Initially, the committee focused on the postoperative period. The PACU nurses worked closely with anesthesia to ensure safe and effective breathing patterns before transfer to the postoperative floor. Patients are identified as a high postoperative respiratory risk by a blueberry wristband and a respiratory-alert medical alert placed on the patient's chart. The respiratory therapy team and the RRT proactively round on these patients, looking at alertness, breathing rate and pattern, as well as oxygen saturation. These initial actions resulted in a 44% reduction of postoperative respiratory events.

MONITORING

Monitoring of the surgical OSA patient includes a complete respiratory assessment, sedation level, positioning (supine position avoided if possible), and oxygen saturation level.[12,26,27] A focused assessment is used while the patient is asleep, watching for signs of OSA such as snoring and periods of stopped breathing.[27] Medications that cause sedation are minimized and use of nonsedating antiemetics and nonopiate analgesia is encouraged.[27] Education of the health care team includes signs and symptoms of OSA, risk factors, and the effects of sedation.[27,28] Adequate communication and hand-off of care includes the risk factors associated with sleep-disordered breathing, assessments (respiratory rate and quality, breath sounds, oxygen saturation), existing conditions, and other factors in care that put the patient at risk.[27,28] Individualized plans of care are based on clinical information and assessment.[28]

Organizations should have policies and procedures in place that regulate standards of care, include documentation guidelines, and hold health care providers accountable for prevention of OSA events.[28] Use of home continuous positive airway pressure (CPAP) or bilevel positive airway pressure (BiPAP) devices should be encouraged and used in both the immediate postoperative period and when the patient is transferred to the floor.[27] CPAP and BiPAP protects the airway by creating a pneumatic splint for the oropharynx.[12]

NEXT STEPS

Our next steps included using a preoperative screening tool and the STOP-Bang questionnaire to identify patients at risk for OSA (**Table 2**). A PACU OSA guideline to standardize care of the of the immediate postoperative patients who are diagnosed or have suspected OSA was created and implemented.

The PACU OSA guideline involves the care of the postoperative OSA patient, including the known CPAP or BiPAP compliant OSA patient, the known CPAP or BiPAP noncompliant patient, and the positive screen for high-risk OSA patient. Known OSA patients are encouraged to bring their own machine. If they are unable, the hospital will provide a machine during their hospitalization. Noncompliant or positive high-risk screened patients follow a similar pathway. If the patient passes the oxygen withdrawal trial, with effective respirations, and no observed apnea, the patient is monitored an additional 2 to 4 hours in PACU.

If the patient fails the oxygen withdrawal trial and/or show signs or symptoms of OSA, the physician will be notified. CPAP or BiPAP will be ordered and the PACU stay will be extended. The anesthesiologist and surgeon will be notified if the patient is noncompliant with CPAP or BiPAP. Possible ICU or intermediate level of care will be ordered, as well as a possible pulmonary consult. If the patient is compliant with CPAP or BiPAP, a trial will be done every 2 hours to monitor for periods of apnea. If the patient has effective respirations, passes the oxygen withdrawal trial, and no additional signs of apnea are seen, transfer to the postoperative floor occurs. Continued failure of the oxygen withdrawal trial, ineffective respirations, and periods of apnea will result in an ICU or intermediate care admission, as well as a pulmonary consult.

SCREENING

OSA that is undiagnosed creates a variety of potential problems for the health care team caring for surgical patients. Undiagnosed and/or untreated OSA surgical patients have higher rates of postoperative complications, are more difficult to intubate, have higher ICU transfer rates, and increased length of stay.[40] Asymptomatic OSA is also associated with increased morbidity and mortality.[41] Prevention of postoperative OSA complications starts with identifying patients who are at risk.[40] Although PSG remains the diagnostic standard for OSA, it is time consuming and expensive. For this reason, Chung and colleagues created the STOP-Bang questionnaire (**Table 3**) that is concise, easy-to-use, and validated in the screening of surgical patients at risk for OSA.[40]

The tool is based on eight items that incorporate four predictive yes-or-no answers and four predictive demographics (S=snore, T=tired, O=observed, P=pressure, B=BMI, a=age=n=neck, g=gender). High risk for OSA is indicated with a score of greater than or equal to three. The STOP questions of the tool are sensitive in detecting surgical patients with moderate to severe OSA. Sensitivity improved when incorporating the Bang portion of the tool.[40,42] The high negative predictive value of the STOP-Bang questionnaire allows for patients who score low to be excluded from the possibility of having moderate to severe OSA.[40] One study validated the STOP-Bang tool and found it to have a sensitivity of 91.7% and a specificity of 63.4% in identifying subjects at high risk for postoperative complications.[43] Another study found that a score of three on the STOP-Bang questionnaire had a sensitivity of 90% and

Table 2
Symptoms and complications or comorbidities of OSA

Symptoms

Excessive daytime sleepiness[14,29]

Excessive or disruptive snoring[14,29]

Gasping for air, snorting breath, waking up to breathe[30]

Periods of apnea during sleep (reported by bed partners)[29]

Morning headaches[29,31]

Irritability, personality changes, depression[8,29]

Difficulty or poor concentration[8,29]

Complications or Comorbidities	Pathophysiology or Prevalence
Hypertension (HTN)	• Chronic elevated sympathetic tone, baroreceptor dysfunction[14] • Risk for developing increases 3-fold[15] • 50%–60% of patients with OSA have HTN[12] • Patients with resistant HTN: 83% had OSA[15]
Cardiovascular Disease (CVD)	• Sympathetic activation, hypoxia or reoxygenation-induced oxidative stress causing vascular inflammation, platelet activation, and deterioration of endothelial function[12,32] • Chronic inflammation contributes to atherosclerosis[33] • OSA contributed to 5-fold increase risk of CVD independent of BMI, systolic or diastolic blood pressure, and smoking[32]
Cardiac Arrhythmias	• Correlates with severity of oxygen desaturation and length of apnea[21] • Sinus bradytachyarrhythmia is most common[21] • Atrial fibrillation and OSA often coexist[34]
Heart Failure	• Increased BMI, atrial fibrillation, HTN, varying intrathoracic pressures due to obstruction[12,34] • Right-sided failure from pulmonary HTN[34] • OSA present in 40% of patients with heart failure[34]
Pulmonary Hypertension	• Hypoxic pulmonary vasoconstriction and remodeling[34] • 17% of patients with OSA[34]
Cerebrovascular Disease	• Hypoxic stress causes vascular inflammation and platelet activation (silent brain infarction), atrial fibrillation often present[33–35] • Inflammation contributes to atherosclerosis[33] • 43%–72% of patients with a stroke have OSA[15]
Diabetes or Metabolic Syndrome	• Increased insulin resistance associated with obesity and HTN[15,36] • OSA adversely affects glucose metabolism, higher insulin secretion and lower insulin sensitivity[37] • Patients with diabetes need to be questioned about OSA[15]
Neurocognitive	• Related to sleep fragmentation or neural damage due to intermittent hypoxia[38] • Decreased cognitive function in areas of attention, learning, memory[38,39] • Major factor in motor vehicle crashes[39]

Table 3	
STOP-Bang questionnaire	
Questions	**Answer**
1. Do you snore loudly? (loud enough to be heard through closed door)	Yes/No
2. Do you often feel tired, fatigued, or sleepy during daytime?	Yes/No
3. Has anyone observed you stop breathing during your sleep?	Yes/No
4. Do you have or are you being treated for high blood pressure?	Yes/No
5. BMI $\geq$35 kg/m^2?	Yes/No
6. Age $\geq$50 y old?	Yes/No
7. Neck Circumference $\geq$40 cm	Yes/No
8. Gender Male?	Yes/No

High Risk of OSA: answering yes to three or more items.
 Low Risk of OSA: answering yes to less than three items.
 Adapted from Chung F, Yegneswaran B, Liao P, et al. STOP questionnaire: a tool to screen patients for obstructive sleep apnea. Anesthesiology 2008;108:774; with permission.

a high positive predictive value of 85% to identify OSA in obese surgical subjects.[44] Chung and colleagues did another study looking at the predictive probabilities of the STOP-Bang questionnaire based on different scores and concluded that a score less than three rules out the risk for OSA.[41] A score of five to eight identifies subjects with increased probability of moderate to severe OSA with the score cut-off of three or more being used for high OSA prevalence surgical subjects. Continued used of a predictive OSA screening tool is essential to identify high-risk patients so that early intervention and treatment can include perioperative precautions to prevent possible harm.[41]

Our hospital's multidisciplinary team implemented changes and process improvements to identify and treat high-risk OSA patients. Over 4 years, the incidence of postoperative respiratory depression complications from oversedation in the hospital has decreased by 53% (**Fig. 1**). Complications decreased by 75% (**Fig. 2**) in the orthopedic patient population. Efforts to identify and proactively treat high-risk patients is ongoing.

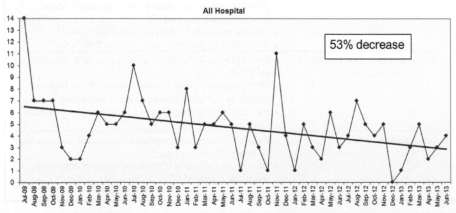

Fig. 1. A significant drop over 4 years of oversedation events in all hospitalized patients due to the work by the Post Operative Respiratory Depression Committee.

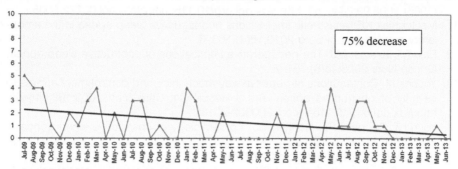

Fig. 2. A reduction of oversedation events in the orthopedic surgery population.

SUMMARY

Untreated or unknown OSA remains a high-risk factor for potential complications in patients undergoing surgical procedures. Having mechanisms in place for the use of validated screening tools, early intervention, goal-directed treatment, and diligent surveillance can be effective in ensuring safe and optimal care of the surgical OSA patient. Post operative respiratory depression and oversedation events can be significantly reduced to improve outcomes for this vulnerable patient population.

REFERENCES

1. Liao P, Yegneswaran B, Vairavanathan S, et al. Postoperative complications in patients with obstructive sleep apnea: a retrospective matched cohort study. Can J Anaesth 2009;56:819–28. http://dx.doi.org/10.1007/s12630-009-9190-y.
2. Hwang D, Shakir N, Limann B, et al. Association of sleep-disordered breathing with postoperative complications. Chest 2008;133(5):1128–34. Available at: http://journal.publications.chestnet.org.
3. Gupta RM, Parvizi J, Hanssen AD, et al. Postoperative complications in patients with obstructive sleep apnea syndrome undergoing hip or knee replacement: a case-control study. Mayo Clin Proc 2001;76(9):897–905. http://dx.doi.org/10.1016/S0025-6196(11)62108-3.
4. Adesanya AO, Lee W, Greilich NB, et al. Perioperative management of obstructive sleep apnea. Chest 2010;138(6):1489–98. http://dx.doi.org/10.1378/chest.10-1108.
5. Memtsoudis S, Liu SS, Ma Y, et al. Perioperative pulmonary outcomes in patients with sleep apnea after noncardiac surgery. Anesth Analg 2011;112(1):113–21. http://dx.doi.org/10.1213/ANE.0b013e3182009abf.
6. Kushida CA, Littner MR, Morgenthaler T, et al. Practice parameters for the indications for polysomnography and related procedures: an update for 2005. Sleep 2005;28(4):499–521.
7. Iber C, Ancoli-Israel S, Chesson AL, et al. The AASM manual for the scoring of sleep and associated events: rules, terminology, and technical specifications. Westchester (IL): American Academy of Sleep Medicine; 2007.
8. Gutierrez C, Brady P. Obstructive sleep apnea: a diagnostic and treatment guide. J Fam Pract 2013;62(10):565–72. Available at: http://jfponline.com.
9. Fogel RB, Malhorta A, White DP. Sleep. 2: pathophysiology of obstructive sleep apnoea/hypopnea syndrome. Thorax 2004;59:159–63. http://dx.doi.org/10.1136/thorax.2003.015859.

10. Ryan CM, Bradley TD. Pathogenesis of obstructive sleep apnea. J Appl Physiol (1985) 2005;99:2440–50. http://dx.doi.org/10.1152/japplphysiol.00772.2005.
11. McGoldrick KE. Anesthetic implications of obstructive sleep apnea in the ambulatory setting. Ambul Surg 2010;16(4):103–6.
12. Paje DT, Kremer MJ. The perioperative implications of obstructive sleep apnea. Orthop Nurs 2006;25(5):291–7.
13. Younes M. Contributions of upper airway mechanics and control mechanisms to severity of obstructive apnea. Am J Respir Crit Care Med 2003;168:645–58. http://dx.doi.org/10.1164/rccm.200302-2010C.
14. Young T, Peppard PE, Gottlieb DJ. Epidemiology of obstructive sleep apnea: a population health perspective. Am J Respir Crit Care Med 2002;165:1217–39. http://dx.doi.org/10.1164/rrcm.2109080.
15. Young T, Skatrud J, Peppard PE. Risk factors for obstructive sleep apnea in adults. JAMA 2004;291(16):2013–6. http://dx.doi.org/10.1001/jama.291.16.2013.
16. Young T, Palta M, Dempsey J, et al. The occurrence of sleep-disordered breathing among middle-aged adults. N Engl J Med 1993;328:1230–5.
17. Pranathiageswaran S, Badr MS, Severson R, et al. The influence of race on the severity of sleep disordered breathing. J Clin Sleep Med 2013;9(4):303–9. Available at: http://dx.doi.org/10.5664/jscm.2572.
18. Eckert DJ, Malhotra A. Pathophysiology of adult obstructive sleep apnea. Proc Am Thorac Soc 2008;5:144–53. http://dx.doi.org/10.1513/pats.200707-114MG.
19. Finkel KJ, Searleman AC, Tymkew H, et al. Prevalence of undiagnosed obstructive sleep apnea among adult surgical patients in an academic medical center. Sleep Med 2009;10:753–8. http://dx.doi.org/10.1016/j.sleep.2008.08.007.
20. Chung SA, Yuan H, Chung F. A systemic review of obstructive sleep apnea and its implications for anesthesiologists. Anesth Analg 2008;107(5):1543–63. http://dx.doi.org/10.1213/ane.0b013e318187c83a.
21. Kaw R, Michota F, Jaffer A, et al. Unrecognized sleep apnea in the surgical patients: implications for the perioperative setting. Chest 2006;129:198–205. Available at: http://journal.publications.chestnet.org.
22. Gay PC. Sleep and sleep-disordered breathing in the hospitalized patient. Respir Care 2010;55(9):1240–54. Available at: http://rc.rcjournal.com/content/55/9/1240.short.
23. Joosten SA, O'Driscoll DM, Berger PJ, et al. Supine position related obstructive sleep apnea in adults: pathogenesis and treatment. Sleep Med Rev 2014;18: 7–17. Available at: http://dx.doi.org/10.1016/j.smrv.2013.01.005.
24. Raw R, Pasupuleti V, Walker E, et al. Postoperative complications in patients with obstructive sleep apnea. Chest 2012;141(2):436–41. http://dx.doi.org/10.1378/chest.11-0283.
25. Pereira H, Xara D, Mendonca J, et al. Patients with a high risk for obstructive sleep apnea syndrome: postoperative respiratory complications. Rev Port Pneumol 2013;19(4):144–51.
26. American Society of Anesthesiologists Task Force on Perioperative Management of patients with obstructive sleep apnea. Practice guidelines for the perioperative management of patients with obstructive sleep apnea: an updated report by the American Society of Anesthesiologists Task Force on Perioperative Management of patients with obstructive sleep apnea. Anesthesiology 2006;104:1081–93.
27. Schreiber P, Bolding DJ. Obstructive sleep apnea: patients at risk. Med Surg Matters 2012;21(5):4–8.
28. Jarzyna D, Jungquist CR, Pasero C, et al. American Society for Pain Management Nursing guidelines on monitoring for opioid-induced sedation and respiratory

depression. Pain Manag Nurs 2011;12(3):118–45. http://dx.doi.org/10.1016/j.pmn.2011.06.008.

29. Doyle DJ. Obstructive sleep apnea and the surgical patient. Anesthesiology News 2010;10–31.

30. Henrichs BM, Walsh RP. Is that snoring something to worry about? Anesthetic implications for obstructive sleep apnea. AANA J 2012;80(5):393–401.

31. Sheldon A, Belan I, Neill J, et al. Nursing assessment of obstructive sleep apnea in hospitalised adults: a review of risk factors and screening tools. Contemp Nurse 2009–2010;34(1):19–33.

32. Peker Y, Hedner J, Norum J, et al. Increased incidence of cardiovascular disease in middle-aged men with obstructive sleep apnea. Am J Respir Crit Care Med 2002;166:159–65. http://dx.doi.org/10.1164/rccm.2105124.

33. Minoguchi K, Yokoe T, Tazaki T, et al. Increased carotid intima-media thickness and serum inflammatory markers in obstructive sleep apnea. Am J Respir Crit Care Med 2005;172:625–30. http://dx.doi.org/10.1164/rccm.200412-16520C.

34. Golbin JM, Somers VK, Caples SM. Obstructive sleep apnea, cardiovascular disease, and pulmonary hypertension. Proc Am Thorac Soc 2008;5:200–6. http://dx.doi.org/10.1513/pats.200708-143MG.

35. Minoguchi K, Yokoe T, Tazaki T, et al. Silent brain infarction and platelet activation in obstructive sleep apnea. Am J Respir Crit Care Med 2007;175:612–7. http://dx.doi.org/10.1164/rccm.200608-1141OC.

36. Barker S. Obstructive sleep apnoea and type 2 diabetes: a wake-up call. J Diabetes Nurs 2011;15(10):372–80.

37. Pamidi S, Wroblewski K, Broussard J, et al. Obstructive sleep apnea in young lean men: impact on insulin sensitivity and secretion. Diabetes Care 2012;35:2384–9. http://dx.doi.org/10.2337/dc12-0841.

38. White DP. Sleep apnea. Proc Am Thorac Soc 2006;3:124–8. http://dx.doi.org/10.1513/pats.200510-116JH.

39. George CF. Sleep apnea, alertness, and motor vehicle crashes. Am J Respir Crit Care Med 2007;176:954–6. http://dx.doi.org/10.1164/rccm.200605-629PP.

40. Chung F, Yegneswaran B, Liao P, et al. STOP questionnaire: a tool to screen patients for obstructive sleep apnea. Anesthesiology 2008;108:812–21.

41. Chung F, Subramanyam R, Liao P, et al. High STOP-Bang score indicates a high probability of obstructive sleep apnea. Br J Anaesth 2012;108(5):768–75. http://dx.doi.org/10.1093/bja/aes022.

42. Lockhart EM, Willingham MD, Abdallah AB, et al. Obstructive sleep apnea screening and postoperative mortality in a large surgical cohort. Sleep Med 2013;14:407–15. Available at: http://dx.doi.org/10.1016/j.sleep.2012.10.018.

43. Vasu TS, Doghramji K, Cavallazzi R, et al. Obstructive sleep apnea syndrome and postoperative complications: clinical use of the STOP-BANG questionnaire. Arch Otolaryngol Head Neck Surg 2010;136(10):1020–4. Available at: http://archotol.jamanetwork.com.

44. Chung F, Yang Y, Liao P. Predictive performance of the STOP-Bang score for identifying obstructive sleep apnea in obese patients. Obes Surg 2013;23:2050–7. http://dx.doi.org/10.1007/s11695-013-1006-z.

Therapeutic Hypothermia After Cardiac Arrest and Return of Spontaneous Circulation: It's Complicated

Ryan Beseda, BSN, RN, CCRN[a], Susan Smith, DNP, RN, ACNS-BC[a],*,
Amy Veenstra, RN, CCRN, CMC[b]

KEYWORDS

- Therapeutic hypothermia • Cardiac arrest • Return of spontaneous circulation
- Resuscitation

KEY POINTS

- Providing evidence-based care to patients with return of spontaneous circulation after a cardiac arrest is a recent complex innovation.
- Once resuscitated patients must be assessed for appropriateness for therapeutic hypothermia, be cooled in a timely manner, maintained while hypothermic, rewarmed within a specified time frame, and then assessed for whether hypothermia was successful for the patient through neuroprognostication.
- There are many potential complications that can arise throughout the therapeutic hypothermia process.
- Nurses caring for therapeutic hypothermia patients must be knowledgeable and prepared to provide care to the patient and family.

On returning to work after lunch, a 63-year-old African-American man with a prior medical history of hypertension, coronary artery disease, and intermittent supraventricular tachycardia collapses. His coworkers immediately begin basic life support. Emergency Medical Services (EMS) were notified immediately, who noted that the patient was receiving quality chest compressions and rescue breaths, on their arrival. The initial cardiac rhythm was determined to be a coarse ventricular fibrillation. A shock of 200 biphasic joules was delivered and the patient returned to a sinus rhythm with a pulse. The patient remained unconscious, and was transferred to the emergency department, while receiving ventilatory support.

The authors have nothing to disclose.
[a] Department of Critical Care Services, Baylor University Medical Center at Dallas, 3500 Gaston Avenue, Dallas, TX 75246, USA; [b] Department of Nursing Administration, Baylor University Medical Center at Dallas, 3500 Gaston Avenue, Dallas, TX 75246, USA
* Corresponding author.
E-mail address: SusanH.Smith@baylorhealth.edu

Innovations in health care have the power to transform safety and cost of care.[1] Protocols are often innovations that drive practices to improve patient care outcomes. The Mild Induced Therapeutic Hypothermia Post-Cardiac Arrest protocol used at Baylor University Medical Center is an innovation in care for patients with return of spontaneous circulation (ROSC) after cardiac arrest. This protocol was developed based on American Heart Association (AHA) guidelines and recommendations from the International Liaison Committee on Resuscitation (ILCOR).[2] Care of ROSC patients is complex and the therapeutic hypothermia protocol helps ensure patients receive evidence-based care each and every time.

An estimated 300,000 people are affected by out-of-hospital cardiac arrest in the United States every year and it is the leading cause of death worldwide. Despite advances in cardiopulmonary resuscitation (CPR) techniques and research, survival rates have not made significant progress in the past 30 years. Overall, survival is 7.6%, unchanged from 1978 through 2008. Survival from cardiac arrest caused by ventricular tachycardia, the subset with the best chances of survival, has only increased to 17.7% from 1980 to 2003.[3] During cardiac arrest the body is acutely deprived of oxygen and vital nutrients, while a buildup of metabolites occurs simultaneously.[3,4] The initial insult, however, is not the only cause of injury during cardiac arrest. Directly after cardiac arrest, on ROSC, begins the phase of "postresuscitation disease."[2]

Post–cardiac arrest syndrome can be broken into distinct categories: post–cardiac arrest brain injury, post–cardiac arrest myocardial dysfunction, and systemic ischemia or reperfusion response. This state is often complicated by a fourth component: the unresolved pathologic process that caused the cardiac arrest.[2] Post–cardiac arrest myocardial dysfunction is characterized by global hypokinesis caused by myocardial stunning and acute coronary syndrome.[2,5] The systemic ischemia/reperfusion response results in systemic inflammatory response syndrome, impaired vasoregulation, increased coagulation, adrenal suppression, impaired tissue oxygen delivery and use, and impaired resistance to infection. The underlying cause of the cardiac arrest often persists past ROSC and can be cardiac, pulmonary, infectious, hypovolemic, toxic, or thrombotic in origin.[2,5,6] Each of these pathophysiologies brings its own list of issues and treatment requirements.[2,5–7] Post–cardiac arrest brain injury presents with impaired cerebrovascular autoregulation, limited cerebral edema, and postischemic neurodegeneration.[2,7] These complications add to the complexity of post–cardiac arrest care.

Research has shown therapeutic hypothermia to be one of the most effective treatments for the pathophysiology of the post–cardiac arrest brain injury associated with post–cardiac arrest syndrome.[2,6,7] The acute event of cardiac arrest and subsequent ROSC can create excitotoxicity, disrupted calcium homeostasis, free radical formation, pathologic protease cascades, and activation of cell-death signaling pathways.[2,6] Prolonged cardiac arrest can also cause failure of cerebral microcirculatory reperfusion despite sufficient cerebral perfusion pressure. This can cause persistent ischemia and small infarctions in some brain regions.[2]

The areas of the brain most affected by cardiac arrest are the hippocampus, cortex, cerebellum, corpus striatum, and thalamus. Hippocampus cornu ammonis pyramidal neurons and cerebellar Purkinje cells, respectively, are the most vulnerable areas to injury during a cardiac arrest.[8] Initial theories behind the benefits of induced mild therapeutic hypothermia were in the reduction of cerebral metabolic rate.[9] However, current research suggests the neuroprotective benefits at the molecular level are in three distinct forms: (1) blocking secondary injury cascades, (2) preventing the loss of endogenous neuroprotectants, and (3) inducing beneficial effects.[10]

Treatment and management of the post–cardiac arrest survivor is based on evidence formed from many years of study. Guidelines from the AHA give providers an algorithm through the required phases of the hypothermia process.[5] These include the following:

- Arrest and ROSC
- Resuscitation and evaluation
- Induction
- Maintenance
- Decooling and rewarming
- 72 hour re-evaluation and neuroprognositication[11]

RESUSCITATION AND EVALUATION

The patient remained unarouseable when he arrived in the emergency department. An advanced airway was placed, a 12-lead electrocardiogram was performed, and initial laboratory studies were drawn. On reviewing the chart and previous admissions, it was discovered the patient also had a history of a drug-eluting stent placed 2 years prior in his mid-circumflex artery. He was a known one pack per day smoker, having smoked for as long as he could remember. He also regularly overindulged in alcohol. Six months prior to this cardiac arrest, the patient had been in our emergency department for hypertension, hypokalemia, hypomagnesmia, and persistent supraventricular tachycardia. He was offered surgical ablation for his dysrhythmia, but chose to manage it medically as an outpatient. He was discharged from that admission with a prescription for atenolol, 50 mg, to be taken once a day and told to follow up with his primary physician within 1 to 2 weeks and a cardiologist within 2 to 4 weeks. During this admission, his initial electrocardiogram was interpreted to be sinus rhythm/sinus tachycardia with mild ischemic ST segment changes of less than 1 mm in the lateral precordial leads. Despite an elevated troponin I on initial laboratory studies, the cardiologist decided against emergent percutaneous coronary intervention (PCI) until the patient demonstrated evidence of neurologic recovery. The patient was evaluated for use of mild hypothermia post-ROSC using the inclusion and exclusion criterion of the protocol (Box 1).

A retrospective study observed there are limited data on the combined use of PCI and therapeutic hypothermia. However, the study concluded primary PCI was associated with a positive patient outcome when used in conjunction with therapeutic hypothermia in ST elevation myocardial infarction patients. This study only included patients with an ST segment elevation of greater than or equal to 1 mm in two or more contiguous leads that received PCI and therapeutic hypothermia together.[12] The 2010 AHA guidelines for CPR and emergency cardiac care state that PCI for patients with a cardiac arrest believed to be cardiac in origin may be reasonable even if the presenting rhythm is non–ST elevation myocardial infarction.[5]

INDUCTION

Initial laboratory work before initiation of therapeutic hypothermia revealed normal potassium and calcium levels. The patient's magnesium level was below the institutional accepted lower limit so it was repleted with 1 g of magnesium sulfate intravenously. The patient's initial creatinine was above what is acceptable for the intensive care unit (ICU) electrolyte replacement protocols so any derangements were repleted more cautiously and only by physician orders.

Complete blood count on admission was normal. Initial coagulation studies showed all values to be within normal limits. The patient received a heparin bolus and heparin infusion intravenously by protocol for acute coronary syndrome. Heparin assays were drawn every 6 hours with the coagulation studies to titrate for the therapeutic window until two consecutive therapeutic values were achieved after which subsequent heparin assays were drawn daily.

An intravenous fentanyl drip titrating for comfort using the Critical-Care Pain Observational Tool was initiated. The patient then received an intravenous midazolam drip titrating for sedation goal using the Richmond Agitation Sedation Scale. Once optimal analgesia and sedation were obtained, the patient received an atracurium bolus intravenously and was started on an atracurium intravenous drip titrated as indicated in the hypothermia protocol. Adequate neuromuscular blockade was monitored with a train-of-four peripheral nerve stimulator. The primary goal was to achieve one or two twitches out of four for the optimal amount of paralysis. Train-of-four was assessed every 15 minutes until the desired paralysis was achieved. Monitoring was then performed every hour until the atracurium drip was stopped and train-of-four was back to baseline.

The patient did not receive any cold saline in the field from the EMS providers. Therapeutic hypothermia was induced in the ICU via an intravenous catheter inserted through the femoral vein cycling cooled saline through a balloon attached to the catheter. Temperature was monitored continuously via a Foley catheter by the hypothermia device. A closed feedback loop continued to cool the patient until target temperature was reached. Cooling was begun 2 hours and 43 minutes after ROSC and target temperature of 33°C was reached 4 hours and 10 minutes later. The total time to target temperature from ROSC was 6 hours and 53 minutes.

The patient's family members were at the bedside on admission to the ICU and were present during the induction of hypothermia. His wife and daughter asked possible causes for his cardiac arrest and were worried that his previous arrhythmias had continued despite his prescribed medication. They were updated regularly to his still critical condition and were educated about the hypothermia protocol. They understood how ill he was and were hopeful therapeutic hypothermia would allow him to live. The chaplain was contacted for support as requested by the family members. Social work was also consulted to initiate contact with the family for support of social needs and discharge planning.

Electrolytes

As part of the therapeutic hypothermia protocol, basic metabolic panels, complete blood cell counts, ionized calcium levels, and serum magnesium levels are drawn every 6 hours. This allows for close monitoring for derangements. Serum calcium, magnesium, phosphorus, and potassium tend to decrease during hypothermia and therefore require constant monitoring and repletion throughout the induction and maintenance phases.[13,14] Electrolytes are excreted in larger quantities during induction and maintenance because of tubular dysfunction and a phenomena known as "cold diuresis" caused by the arteriovenous shunting that increases blood flow to core organs, such as the kidneys.[15] Electrolytes remaining in the body are further depleted by migration into the intracellular spaces caused by increased permeability of cellular membranes during hypothermia.[15,16] The resulting serum electrolyte imbalances must be closely monitored and repleted. Electrolyte imbalances such as these have been shown to cause increased arrhythmias. Magnesium in particular has been shown to be instrumental in decreasing brain injury, myocardial dysfunction, and arrhythmias.[16] Potassium and magnesium replacement protocols are incorporated into the therapeutic hypothermia order set and the AHA recommends keeping serum potassium greater than 3.5 mEq/L.[7]

Box 1
Baylor University Medical Center Mild Hypothermia Inclusion and Exclusion Criteria

Inclusion Criterion (ALL criterion must be met)

Cardiac arrest out of hospital or in-hospital witness, with <15 minutes to first attempt of resuscitation

Negative serum pregnancy test or documentation of hysterectomy for women of childbearing age (50 years or younger)

Cardiac arrest believed to be cardiac origin including asystole, pulseless electrical activity, pulseless ventricular tachycardia, or ventricular fibrillation

Cooling can be initiated in <6 hours from return of spontaneous circulation

<60 minutes from collapse to restoration of spontaneous circulation

Mechanically ventilated

Coma suggested by the following: unable to follow simple commands, does not open eyes to painful stimulus, Glasgow Coma Scale ≤8

Age of 18 years or older

Absolute Exclusion Criterion (NONE of the below criteria can exist for the patient to qualify)

Cause of coma of noncardiac origin (cerebral vascular accident, head trauma, drug overdose, status epilepticus)

Known history of terminal illness before arrest (prearrest life expectancy <6 months)

Major trauma

Sustained life-threatening arrhythmias

Core temperature <30°C (86°F) after return of spontaneous circulation

Systolic blood pressure <90 mm Hg despite fluids and vasopressors

Precautions (physician designation whether to proceed with therapeutic hypothermia if meets criteria below)

Active bleeding or known pre-existing coagulopathy

Known sepsis or systemic infection

Techniques for Achieving Hypothermia

Initiation of hypothermia may begin in the field setting implemented by EMS with saline or Ringer's lactate chilled to 4°C.[11] There are two primary methods used for achieving therapeutic hypothermia. The servomechanism systems used to induce and maintain hypothermia are endovascular machines and surface machines.[11,17] In the endovascular system, the machine operates by chilling normal saline to near or below freezing during induction and cycling it through a balloon attached to a central venous catheter. This patient's catheter was placed in the right femoral vein, although other placement locations are available depending on the type of catheter used. The cooling machine takes the data from the temperature monitoring probes and uses a negative closed feedback loop to titrate the temperature of the saline cycling through the balloon to maintain the target temperature.[17]

A surface cooling device uses gel pads that adhere to the thighs, abdomen, and back. Chilled water is cycled through the pads to bring the patient to target temperature. The machine uses data from core temperature monitoring probes just like the endovascular device to titrate the temperature of the water to maintain the target temperature.[17] Research has suggested that neither device is better than the other in inducing and maintaining hypothermia.[11,17]

Coagulopathies

During cooling, platelets are dysfunctional in their ability to adhere and migrate throughout the body. Coagulation enzyme activity also decreases during hypothermia. This can lead to uncontrollable bleeding. In addition, plasminogen activator inhibitor activity decreases with lower temperatures, decreasing the body's ability to inhibit fibrinolysis. The body then has a hindered ability to create clots and cannot stop itself from breaking down existing ones.[13]

Shivering

The human body fiercely combats any change from normothermia. Temperature sensing ion channels throughout the body feed information to the hypothalamus, the thermostat of the body. Inherent body responses are affected by therapeutic hypothermia. The primary defenses of the body against cold and hypothermia are peripheral vasoconstriction, shunting of blood flow to vital organs, and shivering.[18]

Vasoconstriction and arteriovenous shunting allow oxygen and metabolic body heat to stay within the core organs and preserve them. These autonomic responses are metabolically efficient, unlike shivering, which can more than double the metabolic rate in young fit subjects. Autonomic responses complicate therapeutic hypothermia by preventing or delaying the achievement of target temperature, whereas the twofold increase in metabolic rate caused by shivering is enough to prevent reaching target temperature because few cooling devices can overcome the heat production generated.[18]

Vasoconstriction and arteriovenous shunting are also effective and can slow or overcome surface cooling devices because these methods rely on peripheral blood flow to distribute the cold to the core. The most commonly used way to combat vasoconstriction and blood shunting is general anesthetics, which produce profound arteriolar dilation. Plasma norepinephrine concentrations increase by a factor of seven with only a 1°C to 2°C drop, so general anesthetics work to overcome this.[18]

Chemical paralysis with neuromuscular blocking agents absolutely ceases shivering; however, these should never be used without adequate sedation and analgesia. Without adequate sedation and analgesia before induction of chemical paralysis a "locked in" effect would be created with the potential that the patient could become awake and aware during hypothermia if coma were to cease. Sedation alone has been shown to be singularly ineffective in preventing thermogenesis.[18]

Although not used with this patient, application of a brain function monitoring device is now used at our institution with hypothermia patients who are chemically paralyzed with neuromuscular blocking agents to help determine how well sedated they are.[11,19] This device is also capable of picking up masseter movement, which may represent shivering.[11,19,20] Other medications and methods can be considered to control shivering during therapeutic hypothermia. These include acetaminophen, focal counter-warming, buspirone, meperidine, dexmedetomidine, and clonidine.[11] Assessment of severity of shivering using the Bedside Shivering Assessment Scale is recommended.[20] Incidence of seizures post–cardiac arrest is between 19% and 34%. Full continuous electroencephalogram monitoring is recommended if seizures are suspected.[11]

MAINTENANCE

Once target temperature was achieved, the hypothermia unit kept the patient at 33°C ± 0.2°C for the 18-hour maintenance period. During this time, electrolytes and coagulopathy factors continued to be monitored every 6 hours. An arterial blood gas was obtained approximately 1 hour after the patient had been intubated, and was within normal limits. The patient was started on an insulin infusion protocol to achieve ideal blood glucose levels when his second blood glucose was greater than 200 mg/dL. A chest radiograph on Day 2 of hypothermia demonstrated worsening from his initial admission radiograph and presence of atelectasis. Scheduled prophylactic vancomycin and piperacillin/tazobactam were begun at this time. As with all medications, these antibiotics were dosed by a pharmacist based on the patient's kidney function and presence of therapeutic hypothermia.

Ventilator-associated pneumonia prevention precautions including head of bed elevation to 30 degrees, oral care every 4 hours with chlorhexidine rinse every 12 hours, subglottic suctioning every 12 hours, gastrointestinal, and venous thromboembolism precautions were maintained during his entire time on the ventilator. Foley catheter care was provided daily during bathing and included wiping six inches from the meatus with a chlorhexidine bathing cloth. The femoral central line site and dressing were monitored every shift for intactness. The dressing was changed weekly and as needed. The dressing and six inches of tubing from the insertion site were also wiped with a chlorhexidine bathing cloth daily. A chlorhexidine gluconate disk was placed over the catheter insertion site before the clear, bio-occlusive dressing was applied.

The patient was turned and repositioned every 2 hours. He was placed on a low air loss sleep surface. A dressing to reduce friction and shearing was placed on his sacrum on admission and maintained through his ICU stay. The patient's coagulation studies remained within normal limits. Heparin infusion rates were adjusted throughout the maintenance period to sustain a therapeutic serum concentration. The patient's wife and daughter remained almost constantly at the bedside taking shifts to allow the other to rest or eat. The staff, social work, and chaplain continued to provide support and information to them regularly.

Maintaining Target Temperature

There is no one specific guideline for length of maintenance of the target temperature time. A clinical trial studying cerebellar Purkinje cells in rats post–cardiac arrest showed induced mild hypothermia provided protection of these cells. After cardiac arrest and subsequent ROSC, subjects were randomized into groups of normothermia (37°C ± 1°) and hypothermia (33°C ± 1°) initiated immediately after ROSC, and then at 1, 4, or 8 hours after ROSC and maintained for 24 or 48 hours. The conclusion of this research was that hypothermia exerts its greatest neuroprotective benefit 8 to 24 hours post–cardiac arrest.[8] The AHA recommends therapeutic hypothermia be maintained between 32°C and 34°C for at least 12 and up to 24 hours.[2,6]

Ventilation

Research has shown hyperventilation increases neurodegeneration. An abundance of oxygen in any situation can lead to the production of free radicals. In addition, hyperventilation leading to hypocapnia can cause increased cerebral ischemia.[6] Patients undergoing therapeutic hypothermia produce less carbon dioxide. The solubility of carbon dioxide in blood and body temperature has an inversely proportional relationship. The partial pressure of carbon dioxide decreases as body temperature decreases making hypocapnia easier. Arterial blood gas measurements are used to monitor hyperventilation and hypocapnia, which are both related to free radial formation.[9]

Glucose Management

The order set dictates that an insulin infusion by protocol be started if two blood glucose measurements are greater than 200 mg/dL during the cooling or rewarming phases. Glucose must be closely monitored during therapeutic hypothermia because of the body's decreased rate of glucose metabolism. With the decreased rate of insulin production and decreased tissue sensitivity to insulin throughout the body during hypothermia the results are elevated blood glucose levels. These in turn can cause elevated catecholamines and counterregulation hormones.[13] Alteration of blood glucose homeostasis is associated with an increased ICU stay, an increased morbidity, and worsened patient outcomes. Research has shown wide fluctuations in serum glucose levels cause exacerbation of oxidative stress, enhanced monocyte adhesion, and increased apoptotic cell death. The exact causes behind these phenomena are widely unknown.[21]

In a study of serum glucose levels within the post–cardiac arrest patient population undergoing therapeutic hypothermia researchers found that large variability rather than hyperglycemia alone is an independent risk factor for in-hospital mortality and worse 3-month neurologic recovery. Study patients were started on an insulin infusion and rates were titrated every 4 hours by registered nurses using a written algorithm to keep blood glucose levels between 110 and 150 mg/dL.[21] The AHA recommends keeping blood glucose between 144 and 180 mg/dL.[7]

Perfusion

Adequate tissue perfusion must be maintained at all times during hypothermia. During the induction of hypothermia, arteriovenous shunting makes accurate noninvasive blood pressures difficult to obtain. Placement of an arterial line for blood pressure monitoring is recommended during therapeutic hypothermia.[14] Bradycardia is common during therapeutic hypothermia. Stroke volume normally increases during bradycardia; however, with an injured heart and pre-existing conditions, vasopressors and inotropes are often needed to maintain a mean arterial pressure of greater than 65 mm Hg.[14] The ILCOR consensus on postresuscitation care identified no clinical trials to confirm whether vasopressors or inotropes alone improved survival of post–cardiac arrest patients.[6] However, it is imperative that tissues receive adequate perfusion and oxygenation to maintain viability.

Infection Control

Constant vigilance must be maintained by monitoring for signs and symptoms of infection with the fever suppression of hypothermia. Precautions should be taken before inducing therapeutic hypothermia post-ROSC if the patient has a known systemic infection or sepsis. Fever is an innate response to infection and oversuppression of inflammation and fever associated with infection can lead to negative patient outcomes.[13]

Fever differs from hyperthermia in that it is a reaction to a particular insult and is part of the body's natural inflammatory response. Hyperthermia is when the body temperature rises despite the lack of an internal stimulus. Body temperature is controlled within the anterior hypothalamus in the preoptic area. Hyperthermia can be caused by damage to this area, increased intracranial pressure, or hypothyroidism. The preoptic area of the anterior hypothalamus monitors body temperature by sensing the temperature of the blood perfusing it.[22] A febrile state is begun when this area senses the cytokine interleukin-1.[22,23]

When a monocyte or macrophage encounters an infectious microorganism or cellular products of acute trauma, they release interleukin-1, interleukin-6, and tumor necrosis factor. These three cytokines are collectively referred to as "endogenous pyrogens." A febrile state assists the host defenses of the body by decreasing the virulence and/or killing the invading microorganism. Fever also increases lymphocyte production and promotes movement of lymphocytes by enhancing vascular adhesion molecule expression. A series of historical experiments has shown that suppressing the fever response in otherwise healthy subjects with antipyrogenic medications decreases the serum antibody response and prolongs the duration of physical symptoms in comparison with control groups.[23]

A systematic review and meta-analysis found an increased risk for pneumonia and sepsis in patients treated with therapeutic hypothermia. No increase in other infections was found. There were multiple limiting factors, such as variations of inclusion criteria, time to achieving target temperature, and the length of hypothermia maintenance periods. Other limitations included the lack of data on the incidence of patients with suspected systemic infections at induction of hypothermia.[24] These data would help differentiate between infections that were exacerbated by hypothermia and those that were caused by the suppressive effects of hypothermia. Risks of prophylactic antibiotics in this patient population have not been studied.[13] As with any other critically ill patient, care should be taken to initiate infection-prevention strategies for ventilator-associated pneumonia, catheter-associated urinary tract infection, and central line bloodstream infection.[25]

Skin Care

ICU patients are at risk for skin breakdown from decreased movement caused by sedation and paralysis. There is also decreased perfusion of the skin from arteriovenous shunting during hypothermia resulting in poor oxygenation of skin tissue.[13] To prevent pressure ulcers, guidelines recommend the following[26]:

- Regularly repositioning the patient every 2 hours
- Measuring prealbumin levels on admission and every 7 days
- Maintaining nutrition at 75% or greater of goal caloric intake
- Maintaining adequate glucose control
- Using pressure redistribution surfaces to decrease shear and pressure points
- Daily assessment of skin concentrating on known pressure points

Pharmacology During Therapeutic Hypothermia

Each phase of therapeutic hypothermia affects organ systems differently and therefore affects drug metabolism and transport. More research is needed to understand drug metabolism and transport in patients during hypothermia. Some effects of therapeutic hypothermia on pharmacology are already well known. For example, many transport enzymes and binding sites are temperature dependent and require larger concentrations to be stimulated and achieve the desired effects. This affects pharmacodynamics and pharmacokinetics.[27]

Most medications are given intravenously during therapeutic hypothermia, although some require oral administration. Under normal circumstances, the oral route is usually preferred because of its ease of access and use of the body's natural transport and distribution systems. During hypothermia, trials have shown a decreased absorption rate and prolonged drug profile within the body of drugs given orally. This is believed to be caused by a mild ileus that presents during mild hypothermia. Few studies have evaluated the effects of hypothermia on renal excretion. Those that have been done have not found any changes in excretion or serum concentrations of those drugs historically metabolized and excreted by the kidneys.[27]

The most common organ in drug metabolism and transport is the liver. A large portion of drugs that are metabolized by the liver depend on various isoforms of the cytochrome P (CYP)-450. The most common CYP isoforms involved in drug metabolism are isoforms of the CYP3A, CYP2C, and CYP2D superfamilies. Intravenous medications that rely on the liver for metabolism and extraction have three key limiting factors: (1) drugs with a high hepatic extraction rate rely on blood flow through the liver for excretion, (2) drugs with a low hepatic extraction rate rely on specific CYP isoform functional activity and protein binding for their clearance from the body, and (3) the drug's permeability and solubility across a biologic membrane.[27]

Several trials have evaluated the CYP metabolism of medications during hypothermic states.[27] Two adult studies, one with phenytoin[28] and one with vecuronium,[29] showed elevated serum concentrations of their respective drugs during hypothermia. This phenomena suggests a decreased metabolism, although the effect of these increased concentrations is unknown.[27] In the vecuronium trial, despite the concentrations, response was generally unchanged in the hypothermic state, even though larger than usual doses were used.[29] This created a longer half-life but not a stronger reaction to the drug.[29] Similar studies involving midazolam showed decreased clearance and elevated concentrations despite consistent infusion rates between normothermic and hypothermic groups.[30,31] In one of these studies, a five-fold increase in midazolam serum concentrations was observed.[30] More research is needed to evaluate the biologic permeability of medications across membranes during a hypothermic state and the effect these states have on cellular transporters to understand the effect of larger serum concentrations on patients.[27]

Psychosocial Patient and Family Support

Many families express strong feelings of relief and fear while their loved one is undergoing therapeutic hypothermia. The fear stems from the sight of multiple tubes and machines attached to their loved one's cold, still body. The relief is from the belief that now their loved one is receiving quality, professional assistance. In some cases, the family or friends of the patient were the ones who initiated CPR, which can be traumatic. Seeing them receiving a high level of care may be reassuring.[32]

Families only want honest, pertinent information. They report that they already feel overwhelmed by the situation and by large numbers of visitors and telephone calls. They also state they do not need excess information. The seriousness of the situation is usually understood, so platitudes or false hope are not helpful. They want to know what to expect, what nurses are looking for during monitoring and assessments, and when attempts to awaken the patient will begin.[32]

Waiting throughout the entire hypothermia protocol including the neuroprognostication period is stressful. Care should be taken to openly and honestly inform families that only approximately half of all patients awaken with a positive neurologic outcome.[6,33,34] Fear of the future during this period is normal and acceptable.[32] Preparing the families for all possible scenarios is important.[32,34] Nurses must carefully evaluate the family for stressors and supports. Use of resources, such as chaplains, social work, and palliative care, can be beneficial as the patient progresses through the hypothermia protocol.

REWARMING

After 18 hours at target temperature, rewarming the patient began at a rate of 0.5°C each hour as required by the protocol. The patient remained hemodynamically stable during this period. His potassium level was 4 mEq/L 4 hours prior and throughout rewarming. Magnesium levels held at 1.9 mg/dL and were not repleted during rewarming. Calcium levels were within normal limits immediately prior and during rewarming and did not necessitate repletion either. The patient's coagulation studies stayed within acceptable limits for a patient on intravenous heparin.

Guidelines suggest a rewarming rate between 0.25°C and 0.5°C.[2] Rewarming, also known as decooling, is the time when hemodynamic instability is most commonly seen. Controlled rewarming helps to prevent this from occurring. Fluid boluses and vasopressors may be required during this period of time.[11] There have been no studies that have directly monitored potential benefits or complications of rewarming rates.[12]

A literature review focusing on rewarming rates for different pathophysiologies treated with therapeutic hypothermia identified five studies that examined rewarming rates for cardiac arrest patients. Although no complications were documented as a result of rewarming in any of these studies, this was attributed to the lack of intracranial pressure and brain blood flow monitoring in these studies. In traumatic brain injury and cerebral vascular attack patients, the most common complication from rapid rewarming is intracranial hypertension.[12] The hyperthermia typical of cardiac arrest patients that develops postrewarming and the resulting increase in intracranial pressure from hyperthermia would support this phenomena being true in cardiac arrest patients.

NEUROPROGNOSTICATION

Immediately after extubation, the patient was able to follow simple commands. His wife and daughter were exuberant at his being able to speak and recognize them. His delirium and alcohol screens were positive and he was started on the alcohol withdrawal protocol to control his symptoms. On the first day after extubation, the patient became severely agitated from alcohol withdrawal requiring treatment with lorazepam. This was worrisome to his family and staff provided education to them about alcohol withdrawal and how it was independent of his cardiac arrest. The patient received his last dose of lorazepam on Day 3. At this time, he was awake; alert; and oriented to person, place, time, and situation. Although he had no memories of his cardiac arrest or his time in the ICU he was able to remember events up to that point. Physical, occupational, and speech therapies were provided. He was not deemed to need inpatient rehabilitation after discharge. It seemed that this patient benefitted neurologically from induction of therapeutic hypothermia post-ROSC.

Multiple studies have been completed measuring the success rate of therapeutic hypothermia. A meta-analysis found a need to treat of six echoing the recommendations of the ILCOR. The Hypothermia After Cardiac Arrest trial randomized patients who met criteria to a normothermia or hypothermia protocol. At the 6-month follow-up, 55% of the patients in the hypothermia group showed a positive neurologic outcome as opposed to 39% in the normothermia group, which was statistically significant.[33]

Conventional neurologic prognostication examinations are not able to accurately assess neurologic status in therapeutic hypothermia patients being actively cooled because of the necessary intermittent sedation and paralytics used during therapeutic hypothermia.[35,36] Research suggests that neurologic prognosis as defined by clinical signs, electrophysiologic signs, biochemical tests, and neuroimaging should wait until

72 hours after ROSC before determining whether the patient will recover neurologically.[35] One study showed 24% of patients had a lower quality of life and 20%
continued to experience cognitive impairments after discharge home post–cardiac
arrest.[37]

SUMMARY

*The patient received a left heart catheterization the day after his extubation. There was no
change from previous catheterizations, therefore no interventions were required during the
procedure. After he was off the alcohol withdrawal protocol, he was sent for an automatic internal cardiac defibrillator (AICD) placement and transferred out of the ICU to a telemetry floor.*

*The patient was discharged 2 days after his AICD placement with orders for activity as tolerated,
2 g sodium heart healthy diet. Postdischarge follow-up visits were recommended with his primary physician in 1 to 2 weeks and his cardiologist in 2 to 4 weeks. When he followed up
with his cardiologist 2 weeks after discharge, he was admitted for an elective cardiac ablation
of his mid-right-sided septum for treatment of his intermittent supraventricular tachycardia.
Twenty-three days after his ablation the patient was readmitted when his AICD fired to shock
him out of supraventricular tachycardia. During the admission questionnaire, the patient reported he had quit drinking but continued to smoke at least a pack of cigarettes a day with
no intention to quit. He was strongly encouraged to quit smoking and he was provided with
smoking cessation resources available in his community.*

Health care is a complex adaptive system.[38] It is through the understanding of complex adaptive systems and complexity science that clinicians can make progress toward common goals, such as patient safety. Case studies have the ability to reveal the
complexity of the system and give a better understanding of the elements of the system.[39] Even small details in the care of each patient can have a major impact on survival.[40] Innovations, such as the Mild Induced Therapeutic Hypothermia Protocol, help
to make sense of the complexity of care needed by ROSC patients and ensure care
delivered is evidence-based to meet the individual needs of each patient.

REFERENCES

1. O'Neill GD, Ballard SC, Levie J. Launch pad: creating the business case for innovation. In: Porter-O'Grady T, Malloch K, editors. Innovation leadership: creating
   the landscape of health care. Sudbury (MA): Jones and Bartlett Publishers;
   2010. p. 135–66.
2. Neumar RW, Nolan JP, Adrie C, et al. Post cardiac arrest syndrome: epidemiology, pathophysiology, treatment, and prognositication. Circulation 2008;
   118(23):2452–83.
3. Nichol G, Thomas E, Callaway CW. Regional variation in out-of-hospital cardiac
   arrest incidence and outcome. JAMA 2008;300(12):1423–31.
4. Bernard SA, Buist M. Induced hypothermia in critical care medicine: a review. Crit
   Care Med 2003;31(7):2041–51.
5. O'Connor RE, Brady W, Brooks SC, et al. Part 10: acute coronary syndromes:
   American Heart Association guidelines for cardiopulmonary resuscitation and
   emergency cardiovascular care. Circulation 2010;122(18):S787–817.
6. Morrison L, Deakin C, Morley P, et al. Part 8: advanced life support: 2010 International Consensus on Cardiopulmonary Resuscitation and Emergency Cardiovascular Care Science with Treatment Recommendations. Circulation 2010;122(16):
   S345–421.

7. Peberdy M, Callaway C, Neumar R, et al. Part 9: post-cardiac arrest care: 2010 American Heart Association Guidelines for Cardiopulmonary Resuscitation and Emergency Cardiovascular Care. Circulation 2010;122(18):S768–86.

8. Paine MG, Che D, Li L, et al. Cerebellar purkinje neurodegeneration after cardiac arrest: effect of therapeutic hypothermia. Resuscitation 2012;83(12):1511–6.

9. Warner DS. Definitions and physiologic effects of induced hypothermia. In: Nunnally ME, editor. Therapeutic hypothermia in the ICU. Mount Prospect (IL): Society of Critical Care Medicine; 2010. p. 81–7.

10. Kochanek PM. What is mild therapeutic hypothermia?. In: Nunnally M, editor. Therapeutic hypothermia in the ICU. Mount Prospect (IL): Society of Critical Care Medicine; 2010. p. 89–96.

11. Seder DB, Riker RR. Complications of therapeutic hypothermia after cardiac arrest: does the type of cooling device matter? Crit Care Med 2011;39(3): 582–3.

12. Ronnen M, Le May M, Hibbert B, et al. The impact of therapeutic hypothermia as an adjunctive therapy in a regional primary PCI program. Resuscitation 2012; 84(4):460–4.

13. Nunnally ME. Essentials of the maintenance phase of therapeutic cooling. In: Nunnally ME, editor. Therapeutic hypothermia in the ICU. Mount Prospect (IL): Society of Critical Care Medicine; 2010. p. 29–34.

14. Callaway CW. Additional considerations during induction. In: Nunnally ME, editor. Therapeutic hypothermia in the ICU. Mount Prospect (IL): Society of Critical Care Medicine; 2010. p. 21–7.

15. Polderman KH. Mechanisms of action, physiological effects and complications of hypothermia. Crit Care Med 2009;37(7):S186–202.

16. Polderman KH, Herold I. Therapeutic hypothermia and controlled normothermia in the intensive care unit: practical considerations, side effects, and cooling methods. Crit Care Med 2009;37(12):1101–20.

17. Tomte O, Draegni T, Mangschau A, et al. A comparison of intravascular and surface cooling techniques in comatose cardiac arrest survivors. Crit Care Med 2011;39(3):443–9.

18. Sessler DI. Thermoregulatory defense mechanisms. Crit Care Med 2009;37(7): S203–10.

19. Barr J, Fraser GL, Puntillo K, et al. Clinical practice guidelines for the management of pain, agitation and delirium in adult patients in the intensive care unit. Crit Care Med 2013;41(4):263–306.

20. Badjatia N, Strongilis E, Gordon E, et al. Metabolic impact of shivering during temperature modulation: the bedside shivering assessment scale. Stroke 2008; 39:3242–7.

21. Cueni-Villoz N, Devigili A, Delodder F, et al. Increased blood glucose variability during therapeutic hypothermia and outcome after cardiac arrest. Crit Care Med 2011;39(10):2225–31.

22. Lorin MI. Fever in critically ill patients. Semin Pediatr Infect Dis 2000;11(1):13–8.

23. Cannon JG. Perspective on fever: the basic science and conventional medicine. Complement Ther Med 2013;21:S54–60.

24. Geurts M, Macleod MR, Kollmar R, et al. Therapeutic hypothermia and the risk of infection: a systematic review and meta-analysis. Crit Care Med 2014;42: 231–42.

25. Barnes S. Infection prevention and "PLUS" measures toolkit. Kaiser Permanente; 2013. Available at: http://nursingpathways.kp.org/national/quality/infectioncontrol/ toolkit/index.html. Accessed March 29, 2014.

26. Carino G, Ricci D, Bartula D, et al. The HAPU bundle: a tool to reduce the incidence of hospital acquired pressure ulcers in the intensive care unit. Int J Nurs Sci 2012;2(4):34–7.
27. Poloyac SM. Pharmacologic considerations in the patient undergoing therapeutic hypothermia. In: Nunnally ME, editor. Therapeutic hypothermia in the ICU. Mount Prospect (IL): Society of Critical Care Medicine; 2010. p. 35–40.
28. Iida Y, Nishi S, Asada A. Effect of mild therapeutic hypothermia on phenytoin pharmacokinetics. Ther Drug Monit 2001;23:192–7.
29. Caldwell JE, Heier T, Wright PM, et al. Temperature-dependent pharmacokinetics and pharmacodynamics of vecuronium. Anesthesiology 2000;92:84–93.
30. Fukuoka N, Aibiki M, Tsukamoto T, et al. Biphasic concentration change during continuous midazolam administration in brain-injured patients undergoing therapeutic moderate hypothermia. Resuscitation 2004;60:225–30.
31. Hostler D, Zhou J, Tortorici MA, et al. Mild hypothermia alters midazolam pharmacokinetics in normal healthy volunteers. Drug Metab Dispos 2010;14:781–8.
32. Holm MS, Norekval TM, Falun N, et al. Partners' ambivalence towards cardiac arrest and hypothermia treatment: a qualitative study. Nurs Crit Care 2012;17(5):231–8.
33. Zanotti-Cavazzoni S. Who should be cooled? Adult patients. In: Nunnally ME, editor. Therapeutic hypothermia in the ICU. Mount Prospect (IL): Society of Critical Care Medicine; 2010. p. 1–8.
34. Harden J. Take a cool look at hypothermia. Nursing 2011;41(9):46–51.
35. Zanotti-Cavazzoni S. Neurologic prognostication in the era of therapeutic hypothermia. In: Nunnally ME, editor. Therapeutic hypothermia in the ICU. Mount Prospect (IL): Society of Critical Care Medicine; 2010. p. 47–52.
36. Rundgren M, Karlsson T, Nielsen N, et al. Neuron specific enolase and S-100β as predictors of outcome after cardiac arrest and induced hypothermia. Resuscitation 2009;80(7):784–9.
37. Wachelder EM, Moulaert VR, van Heugten C, et al. Life after survival: long term daily functioning and quality of life after an out-of-hospital cardiac arrest. Resuscitation 2009;80(5):517–22.
38. Rogers EM. Diffusion of innovations. 5th edition. New York: Free Press; 2003.
39. Anderson RA, Crabtree BF, Steele DJ, et al. Case study research: the view from complexity science. Qual Health Res 2005;15(5):669–85.
40. Lindberg C, Nash S, Lindberg C. On the edge: nursing in the age of complexity. Bordentown (NJ): PlexusPress; 2008.

Open Access in the Critical Care Environment

Tabitha South, MSN, RN[a,b],*, Brigette Adair, BSN, RN, CCRN, NE-BC[c]

KEYWORDS

- Open access • Open visitation • ICU visiting • Critical care • Family satisfaction
- Nurse perception and attitudes • ICU diary

KEY POINTS

- A focus on patient and family–centered care has led to an increase in open access in the critical care environment.
- Some hospitals have instituted open access with success, whereas others continue to struggle with the health care team opinion that open access could interfere with patient care.
- Evidence-based practice as well as patient satisfaction supports the need for open access in critical care environments.
- It is imperative that families and health care teams have collaborative discussions to decide what type of visitation best meets the needs of the patients.
- Keeping a diary of the events in the intensive care unit can help prevent posttraumatic stress disorder in patients.

INTRODUCTION

Critical care units, also referred to as intensive care units (ICU), are high-stress, fast-paced environments in which critically ill patients are closely monitored for changes in their conditions. Patients in critical care settings experience a gamut of physical and emotional insults that can negatively affect their perceptions of care. In addition, families of patients in the ICU also experience the peripheral impact of a severe illness, which includes fear, anxiety, and stress among other physical and emotional symptoms. Families may refer to anyone who is identified as either a relative, close friend, or significant other. In recent years, there has been an increased focus on the importance of patient and family–centered care. In addition, patients and families have become

The authors have nothing to disclose.
[a] Baylor Regional Medical Center at Grapevine, Grapevine, TX, USA; [b] Medical Surgical Services, Medical Center of Plano, 3901 West 15th Street, Plano, TX 75075, USA; [c] 4 Roberts Intensive Care Unit, Baylor University Medical Center at Dallas, 3500 Gaston Avenue, Dallas, TX, USA
* Corresponding author. Medical Surgical Services, Medical Center of Plano, 3901 West 15th Street, Plano, TX 75075.
E-mail address: tabnderrick@gmail.com

more knowledgeable and have higher expectations regarding their involvement in the care continuum. Along with this increased involvement, family members often provide support and resources for the patients. Hospitals need to recognize the importance of family involvement. The transition to open access in the critical care environment requires health care teams to communicate openly and work as collaborative teams to change unit-based cultures. This article includes a discussion of current findings regarding the transition to open access and some steps that have been taken by various units, hospitals, and health care systems to change the long-standing critical care culture.

SUMMARY/DISCUSSION

The impact of a critical care unit stay on patients and families is severe and is typically given a negative connotation as a result. When patients are admitted to critical care units, they are generally the sickest patients in the facility and require close monitoring and frequent interventions. In the ICU, patients are commonly sedated or even paralyzed and are unable to advocate for their own care. In the past, and currently in some units, ICU patients are kept behind locked doors and families are able to visit for a limited amount of time at intervals throughout the patients' stays. However, this model is unsustainable in the era of patient and family–centered care. More than a decade ago, Hinckle and colleagues[1] reported that, "the Institute of Medicine strongly recommended that healthcare delivery systems become more patient centered, which in ICUs translates into increased family involvement." Henneman and Cardin[2] stated that, "Family-centered care is care that demands a collaborative approach to care in which all members of the team support and value this philosophy." When family members are forced to be separated from their loved ones because of institutional policies, the negative effects on family members of patients in critical units can be exacerbated.

In addition, effective January 2011, Centers for Medicare and Medicaid Services required hospitals to have open access to a primary support person with a goal to move toward patient-centered care. Patient-centered care includes involving patients and/or families in all aspects of care to create ideal care experiences through all the stages of their hospitalizations.

PROBLEM

Patients who are in critical care units and their families often experience a decreased ability to cope caused by the severity of the illness and the impact of that illness on coping. Common psychological responses of patients and family members include anxiety, stress, and a potential lack of trust caused by the uncertainty of the situation. Certain situations, such as restriction of visitation, can contribute to a negative psychological response that is likely to have a negative impact in the healing environment. In contrast, nurses perceive that presence of families can interfere with nursing care and that the emotional involvement contributes to the stress and strain on the patients.

REVIEW OF LITERATURE

At Baylor Health Care System, open access in critical care units has become an expectation with the goal of providing safe passage of care to all patients. The framework for open access is supported by the system Professional Nursing Practice Model, which is adapted from the American Association of Critical-Care Nurses Synergy Model. In this model (**Fig. 1**),[3] the needs of patients are addressed using evidence-

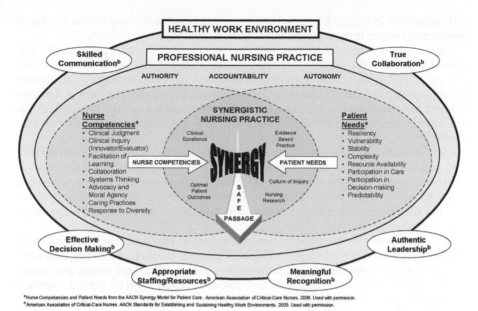

Fig. 1. Baylor Health Care System Professional Nursing Practice Model. (*From* Bradley D, Dixon JF. Staff nurses creating safe passage with evidence-based practice. Nurse Clin N Am 2009;44:71–81. Copyright © Baylor University Medical Center; with permission.)

based practice and research as well as appropriate bedside leader competencies. In critical care patients, there is vulnerability, both emotional and physical. The physical illness component has always been readily addressed by the skilled providers who care for the patients, but the emotional component, which includes a loss of control and often an inability to participate in care and decision making, has not always been fully addressed. This emotional component is the area in which families of patients can potentially fill a void, if allowed. In the traditional model of restricted visitation in critical care, family members often struggle for the ability to see their loved ones for just 1 more minute. They are often overwhelmed by the environmental stimuli of the ICU setting in addition to the altered states in which they are seeing their family members. In this overwhelmed state, it is difficult to ask questions and advocate for the patients in the beds. Aro and colleagues[4] wrote that, "Meeting the needs of family members of critically ill patients should be emphasized. Visiting times should be flexible, and patients and their families should be involved in the decision-making process."

CASE STUDY

A quantitative and qualitative analysis was performed to evaluate family satisfaction in the ICU setting.[5] Key themes, including respect and compassion shown to families, participation of families, and ICU environment were identified as opportunities for improvement.[5] Each of these areas of opportunities provides further support for inclusion of patient-centered care in the critical care environment. In this single-center study, respect and compassion shown to families was an area of great concern in both the quantitative and qualitative data. The study "…also found that compassion and emotional support are important, particularly in the decision-making process. Anxiety and depression are frequent and particularly high in families of nonsurviving

ICU patients."[5] In addition, "shared decision making—the primary model for family participation needs to be adapted to families' needs."[5]

Another key theme besides respect and compassion is the ICU environment. Hospitals address the need to improve effective patient and family–centered care and patient safety by adapting the physical environment and/or adapting the model of care used to manage critically ill patients. The design and development of the environment of a health care facility has a direct impact on patient safety.[6] One design that has seen some success in recent years is the acuity adaptable or universal bed model.[7,8]

A unit or facility that uses an acuity adaptable design for its patients is able to provide care for patients of various levels of acuity in the same room. Each room is capable of caring for patients who require critical care, step-down, observation, and acute care.[9,10] Having acuity appropriate care brought to patients instead of the patients having to go to the care is one way this model supports and encourages patient-centered care.[7,8]

As a result of this model, patients are able to stay in the same room for their entire stay and this can have a significant impact on patients, families, physicians, and staff. Many hospitalized patients experience severe stress related to their illness and related treatments, but, in typical models of care, stress is exacerbated by patient transfer.[9] This increased stress can lead to decreased information processing by patients, which in turn can result in increased demands on the staff.[9] By allowing patients to stay in the same room, the stress of transfer is removed and, as a result, there is an increased sense of control over the environment, which contributes to patients' perception that they are more involved in their plans of care.[9] In addition, consistency of staff allows patients and families to increase rapport building with the care compared with a traditional model involving multiple hand-offs of care. By allowing the patients to stay in the same place reduces the burden on families to find the patients because they always know where the patients will be. The same can be observed in physicians, who have a reduced burden in finding the patients. In addition, because the nursing care is brought to the patients and the same staff work with the same patients, there is an opportunity for nurses and health care providers to build rapport with staff, patients, and families and to improve the focus on patient and family–centered care.[7,8]

Nursing perception and attitude are important factors in consideration of family visitation. In 1 medical ICU that was studied, nurses' perception was that open visitation could lead to increased risk of infection for the patients; interference with the patients' treatment, thereby increasing teams' workloads; increase in patients' stress levels; increased stress levels for patients' family members; and violation of patient privacy.[11] The research shows no solid scientific basis for restricting access for visitors.[11] On the contrary, opening critical care allows families to play an active role in treatment and does not create problems for patients.[11] Restricting visiting in critical care is not caring, compassionate, or necessary.

In Europe, many ICUs have restricted visiting policies. Too many visits are thought to be to the patient's detriment and to interfere with patient care. However, an open visiting policy seems to be more suited to patient and family needs. **Table 1** shows the advantages and disadvantages of an open visiting policy.[12]

Successful implementation of open visiting policies depends on the nurses' attitude to open visitation. In a Belgian study involving 30 ICUs in 17 hospitals a total of 531 nurses completed a questionnaire exploring their views on visitation.[12] The survey asked ICU nurses about their beliefs and attitudes about visitation, visiting hours, and open visiting policies in a critical care setting. The study concluded that ICU nurses were skeptical about an open visiting policy.[12]

Table 1		
The advantages and disadvantages of an open visiting policy		
	Advantages of Open Visiting Policy	Disadvantages of Open Visiting Policy
For patients	Increased patient satisfaction Promoting patient recovery by reducing stress Positive psychological effect Positive effects on vital signs	Patients not getting enough rest Nurses have less time for the patients Harmful physiologic consequences
For families	Decreased stress Decreased anxiety Able to visit whenever they want Better informed	Family members become exhausted and feel obligated to stay

For health
  care workers
	Increased job satisfaction from
	  family members' positive
	  feedback
	Families as a helpful support
	  structure, facilitating
	  communication and increased
	  educational opportunities
	Enhance nursing care delivery
	  because of having more
	  information from families
	Better working relationship
	  between staff and families
		Families want continuous information
		Increased nursing stress
		Nurses being distracted
		Closer emotional involvement

Data from Berti D, Ferdinande P, Moons P. Beliefs and attitudes of intensive care nurses toward visits and open visiting policy. Intensive Care Med 2007;33:1060–5.

Research has also indicated that nurses claimed that visiting interfered with nursing care and that the emotional involvement with families produced stress and strain for the patients.[13] The perception of nurses is that the primary concern is for the patients but that the families' needs must also be met. Review of the literature indicates that although nursing staff identify that families at times can be a contributor to stress, benefits of open visitation outweigh the risks.[13] Research has consistently shown that unrestricted visitation results in increased family satisfaction, patient reports of more happiness and less anxiety, and improved communication between families and caregivers.[13]

Despite the positive findings, open visitation does not mean visitation without guidelines. For open visitation to be successful, a collaborative discussion needs to occur among patients, families, and health care teams. Hospital and unit visitation policies should routinely be reviewed and revised in a shared governance council (ie, ICU Partnership Council) to ensure opportunities for nurses to individualize visitation to meet the patients' and families' needs as well as those of the health care teams.[14]

Patient satisfaction is another area in which open visitation can have a positive impact. Research has been conducted in different hospitals using an acuity adaptable model in 1 or more units and assessing patient satisfaction scores, such as the Press Ganey survey, as an outcome measure.[8] In one recent study, a Cardiac Universal bed model was used and patient satisfaction as a result was at the 99th percentile for more than 2 years in both the inpatient departments and emergency department.[8] In another study, a urologic acuity adaptable model was implemented and in the first 2 years maintained the highest overall patient satisfaction of the facility as measured by Press Ganey.[9] A similar study was conducted at a separate facility and found that patients were 100% satisfied with this model of care compared with the traditional model of care.[15] The review of this literature suggests that these models may help increase patient satisfaction in the ICU.

In some health care organizations the Critical Care Family Satisfaction Survey (CCFSS), which includes both quantitative and qualitative data, has been used to measure family members' satisfaction in critical care.[16] In one pilot study in an ICU in Sweden, the summary of the results from the CCFSS indicated that flexible visiting hours were valued by family members. The most common source of stress for family members included uncertainty about prognosis and outcome.[16] This survey provides more timely feedback pertinent in the critical care area.

Family visitation could also have a positive impact on the patients' recovery by decreasing post–intensive care syndrome (PICS). An increasing number of ICU patients who survive develop mental, cognitive, and physical impairments referred to as PICS.[17] In 3 studies, including 2 randomised controlled trials, medical staff and families kept a daily diary, including both pictures and text, for each patient during the ICU stay.[17] The patients were assessed at various time intervals after ICU discharge, and anxiety and depression symptoms decreased significantly. The research supports the use of ICU diaries to reduce mental health complications related to ICU survival.[17] In another study, patients keeping a diary while in the ICU showed the best evidence for reducing symptoms of posttraumatic stress disorder (PTSD).[18] The ICU diary was used to document symptoms and events. Once patients had been transferred out of the ICU, they were encouraged to read and then to discuss the events written in the diary in the hope that it may help to prevent PTSD.[18] The ICU staff found it hard in this study to update the diaries; therefore, it may be more effective if families updates the diaries. This experience supports open access for the primary support family member.

SUMMARY/IMPLICATIONS FOR PRACTICE

Much of the focus of this article has been on the ability of family members to have access to their loved ones in critical care environments, but a key rationale is to enable patients to have open access to those they need for support. Although many nurses, units, and hospitals have concerns regarding the ability for nurses to continue to provide high-quality care with families present, nurses who have adopted this model have found little to no negative impact.

Patient and family–centered care gives patients and families the opportunity to be informed and involved in decision making as valued members of the health care team. Actively involving patients in their care improves the quality of care and improves satisfaction for patients and care givers. A patient and family–centered model of care also guides and supports those providing care in attending to their patients' and families' physical and emotional needs, and maintaining or improving their quality of life to the greatest extent possible (**Box 1**).

Every health care system and hospital has the ability to develop and sustain effective partnerships with patients and families to enhance quality, safety, and the experience of care. ICU units that effectively incorporate patient and family–centered care have increased recruitment and retention of staff, increased satisfaction of patients and families, improved quality of care, and improved outcomes, while decreasing anxiety and stress for patients and families, decreasing lengths of stay, and decreasing overall cost. "Therefore, family involvement and visitation policy should be flexible for patients and their families and be related to the patients' best interest."[4]

Box 1
Open access in critical care is an essential aspect of an increased focus on patient and family centeredness. Patient and family–centered inpatient units consistently have these features

- Shorter lengths of stay
- Higher-than-average overall patient satisfaction scores
- Increased staff retention
- Enhanced staff recruitment
- Decreased emergency department return visits
- Fewer medication errors

Adapted from Charmel P, Frampton S. Building the business case for patient-centered care. Healthc Financ Manag 2008;62:80–5; with permission.

REFERENCES

1. Hinkle J, Fitzpatrick E, Oskrochi G. Identifying the perception of needs of family members visiting and nurses working in the intensive care unit. J Neurosci Nurs 2009;41:85–91.
2. Henneman E, Cardin S. Family-centered critical care: a practical approach to making it happen. Crit Care Nurse 2002;22:12–9.
3. Bradley D, Dixon JF. Staff nurses creating safe passage with evidence-based practice. Nurs Clin N Am 2009;44:71–81.
4. Aro I, Pietila A, Vehvilainen-Julkunen K. Needs of adult patients in intensive care units of Estonian hospitals: a questionnaire survey. J Clin Nurs 2012;21: 1847–58.
5. Schwarzkopf D, Behrend S, Skupin H, et al. Family satisfaction in the intensive care unit: a quantitative and qualitative analysis. Intensive Care Med 2013;39: 1071–9.
6. Cesario S. Designing health care environments: part 1: basic concepts, principles, and issues related to evidence-based design. J Contin Educ Nurs 2009;40:280–8.
7. Brown K, Galland D. Impacting patient outcomes through design: acuity adaptable care/universal room design. Crit Care Nurse 2006;29:326–41.
8. Winter M, Tjiong L, Houston S. The challenges and rewards of the cardiac universal bed model. Nurs Manag 2011;42:46–50.
9. Annonio J, Graham J, Ross R. Using an acuity-adaptable unit for urologic services. Urol Nurs 2010;30:223–7.
10. Ritchey T, Stichler J. Determining the optimal number of patient rooms for an acute care unit. J Nurs Adm 2008;38:262–6.
11. Giannini A. Open intensive care units: the case in favour. Minerva Anestesiol 2007;73:299–306.
12. Berti D, Ferdinande P, Moons P. Beliefs and attitudes of intensive care nurses toward visits and open visiting policy. Intensive Care Med 2007;33:1060–5.
13. Whitton S, Pittiglio LI. Critical care open visiting hours. Crit Care Nurse 2011; 34(4):361–6.
14. Simon S, Phillips K, Badalamenti S, et al. Current practices regarding visitation policies in critical care units. Am J Crit Care 1997;6(3):210–7.
15. Clark E, Roberts C, Traylor KC. Cardiovascular single-unit stay: a case study in change. Am J Crit Care 2004;13:406–9.

16. Karlsson C, Tisell A, Engstrom A, et al. Family members' satisfaction with critical care: a pilot study. Nurs Crit Care 2011;16(1):11–8.
17. Parker AM, Sricharoenchai T, Needham DM. Early rehabilitation in the intensive care unit: preventing impairment of physical and mental health. Curr Phys Med Rehabil Rep 2013;1:307–14.
18. Mehlhorn J, Freytag A, Schmidt K, et al. Rehabilitation interventions for postintensive care syndrome: a systematic review. Illinois: Society of Critical Care Medicine and Lippincott Williams & Wilkins; 2014. p. 1–9.

Review of Evidence About Family Presence During Resuscitation

Sonya A. Flanders, MSN, RN, ACNS-BC, CCRN[a,]*,
Jessica H. Strasen, BSN, RN, CCRN[b]

KEYWORDS

- Family presence during resuscitation • Family-witnessed resuscitation
- Family-centered care • Patient-centered care • Resuscitation

KEY POINTS

- Despite research documenting family presence during resuscitation (FPDR) is unlikely to cause psychological distress to families and may be helpful to them, the practice remains controversial in many settings.
- Being present during a loved one's resuscitation should be offered as an option to family, ideally in alignment with the patient's wishes, and with a designated family support person.
- Health care providers (HCPs) generally are less supportive of FPDR than patients and families, and levels of support vary by geographic region and culture.
- Variations in practice regarding FPDR may lead to inequitable patient care. Patients, families, and HCPs deserve to receive and give evidence-based care related to FPDR.
- HCP education about FPDR, policies or guidelines, and experience with FPDR tend to increase HCP support for the practice.

INTRODUCTION

A desirable attribute of nursing practice is to provide patient care based on evidence. Sometimes personal attitudes, opinions, traditions, and beliefs also influence nursing decisions and actions, as does the context of the practice environment. Care of the dying patient and his or her family is a complex, emotionally charged situation susceptible to personal attitudes of nurses and other health care providers (HCPs). Patients nearing the end of life require skilled nursing care at all times, but perhaps more so when death is unexpected and resuscitation is attempted.

Disclosure Statement: The authors have no significant relationships to disclose.
[a] Center for Learning Innovation and Practice, Baylor Scott & White Health, 2001 Bryan Street, Suite 600, Dallas, North Texas 75201, USA; [b] 4 Truett Medical ICU, Baylor University Medical Center at Dallas, 3500 Gaston Avenue, Dallas, TX 75246, USA
* Corresponding author.
E-mail address: sonyaf@baylorhealth.edu

Crit Care Nurs Clin N Am 26 (2014) 533–550
http://dx.doi.org/10.1016/j.ccell.2014.08.010
0899-5885/14/$ – see front matter © 2014 Elsevier Inc. All rights reserved.

To guide nurses and interdisciplinary colleagues, medical aspects of care during resuscitation are outlined in evidence-based basic and advanced cardiac life support (ACLS) guidelines.[1,2] Resuscitation guidelines facilitate shared expectations and collaborative workflow among members of health care teams. Technical aspects of resuscitation such as cardiopulmonary resuscitation (CPR), advanced airway management, electrical therapies, and medication administration have been widely adopted and generally agreed upon. Resuscitation activities may also involve ethical considerations, including whether to allow family presence (FP) at resuscitation, an issue about which resuscitation team members may disagree. Although several organizations[3–7] support offering the option of family presence during resuscitation (FPDR), implementation remains controversial. The problem is controversy leads to practice variation, so some families are offered this option while others are not. Inconsistent practice opens the door for inequitable patient care, and also poses a risk to the health care team as inconsistencies may lead to confusion, tension, or overt conflict between HCPs. Given the potential consequences, nurses and others may benefit from examining what is known about FPDR, including factors that hinder and help effective implementation, so as to best care for patients, families, and one another. This article presents relevant research on attitudes about FPDR, interventions to help change practice, and the authors' experience with a project to implement FPDR in a medical intensive care unit (MICU). This knowledge can be used to empower nurses to transfer evidence into practice.

BACKGROUND

FPDR remains a popular topic in contemporary health care literature. FPDR means family members are offered the option to witness any portion of resuscitation efforts on their loved one. Presence may range from allowing family members to touch or speak to the patient to having them passively observe without patient interaction. Offering FPDR as an option means the choice is offered devoid of coercive behavior intended to promote or discourage a specific decision. The optional aspect is important because FPDR may not be desirable for everyone. The term family, historically defined as one's legal relatives, has expanded. Besides legal relatives, the Joint Commission's definition includes friends or others who provide support to the patient as family.[8] Similarly, the American Association of Critical Care Nurses (AACN) defines family as including relatives and significant others who have an established relationship with the patient.[4] Clarifying who is considered family should be part of dialogue about FPDR to minimize misunderstandings.

The first article addressing FPDR was published more than 25 years ago, when researchers found most families wished to be present during resuscitation, and most staff surveyed endorsed FPDR.[9] Although there was a paucity of research over the following decade, interest in FPDR later resurfaced. Today there is a substantial body of literature surrounding the practice.

REVIEW OF EVIDENCE ABOUT FAMILY PRESENCE DURING RESUSCITATION

Available evidence can add objectivity to the creation of well-informed practice recommendations. The literature contains reports about HCP, patient, and public attitudes about and experiences with FPDR, offering viewpoints from key stakeholder groups. In addition, effects of various interventions used to change practice have been explored. Research findings about attitudes and experiences can guide planning and implementation of FPDR, and help to promote buy-in of interprofessional staff and organizational leaders.

The Origins of Research

The landmark study about FPDR continues to be cited in contemporary literature, and some issues addressed then remain controversial today. Researchers were inspired to learn more about having families attend resuscitation events after a chaplain-administered survey revealed 72% of family members wished they had been present during resuscitation efforts.[9] As a result, they conducted a program in one Michigan hospital's emergency department (ED), allowing selected family members to attend resuscitations, then surveyed families and staff. Results indicated most family members would want to attend a family member's resuscitation again, approximately one-third considered it their right, and the majority believed it aided their grieving and was beneficial to their dying family member. Of staff respondents, 81% had been with family in the resuscitation room and 30% thought anxiety had hampered their activities, but 71% still endorsed FPDR. Researchers concluded there were no data to support denying FPDR, found no difference in resuscitation attempts whether family was present or not, and indicated that no families had interfered with resuscitation. Having a supportive, dedicated staff member such as a chaplain or nurse to assist the family was noted as a crucial requirement for the success of an FPDR program.[9] This study provided new insight into FPDR and challenged opposing arguments, offering a foundation for additional research into an unexplored practice.

An anecdotal report from the same hospital described how, after 9 years of allowing FPDR, there had been no instances of interference with resuscitation efforts.[10] The investigators said, "with 9 years of experience in facilitating acceptance of death and grieving by this method, it is hard for us to understand that this practice is seldom considered."[10(p106)] Nonetheless, FPDR remains controversial.

Health Care Provider Attitudes About Family Presence

Further research has examined FPDR from the viewpoints of HCPs (**Box 1** provides a summary). Some research has revealed divided opinions between health care disciplines. For example, investigators gathered opinions from members of the Emergency Nurses Association (ENA) and the American Association for the Surgery of Trauma (AAST) about FP during trauma resuscitation after nurses in one trauma center attempted to implement a policy supporting FPDR.[11] Group opinions differed significantly about which procedures family should be permitted to observe, with ENA members voicing greater support than the physicians. Nurses believed family had a right to be present, and would rather be present themselves if their family member needed resuscitating. By contrast, AAST members thought FP would interfere with resuscitation, increase providers' stress levels, and raise litigation risk. Researchers expressed concerns about patient confidentiality and safety of trauma team members from potentially violent family members, concluding a policy allowing FPDR would create disharmony between team members.[11]

Another survey was conducted with a sample predominantly comprised of physicians, with a smaller number of nurses and other allied health professionals.[12] Most respondents did not support FPDR, although nurses again were more likely to support FPDR than others. Levels of support varied regionally across the United States, with Midwesterners more likely to endorse FPDR. Reasons for disapproval included worries of psychological trauma to family, medicolegal concerns, HCP performance anxiety, and fear of family distracting the resuscitation team.[12]

In a study seeking only nurses' opinions, acute care nurses and ENA members in New Jersey were queried about attitudes regarding FPDR and invasive procedures (IP).[13] The survey was completed by 193 registered nurses (RNs) and 15 licensed

---

Box 1
Perceptions of health care providers (HCPs) about FPDR

Concerns

Concerns affecting patients and families

- Psychological distress to family
- Organizational culture may conflict with patient/family culture
- Compromised patient confidentiality
- Interference with patient resuscitation
- Inadequate space for family
- Risk of injury to family
- May cause prolonged resuscitation
- Family may be upset by things said by resuscitation team
- Family may misinterpret activities during resuscitation

Concerns affecting the health care team

- Create discord between HCPs
- Medicolegal risk
- Distracting to resuscitation team
- Risk to safety of resuscitation team
- Need to abide by legal and forensic rules
- Increased staff needed for FPDR and may increase costs
- Stress for staff related to be observed
- Interference with teaching of residents

Benefits

- Improves communication between staff and family
- Staff could explain resuscitation to family
- Facilitates family's acceptance of death
- Provides family a sense of control
- Facilitates family's grieving process
- Relatives could see everything possible was done
- Family could help decide when to terminate resuscitation efforts
- Enhanced personhood of the patient
- Family help the patient

Data from Refs.[11–13,15–17,21–32]

---

practical nurses (LPNs). Although 58% indicated that FPDR interfered with job performance, 56% would want to attend resuscitation of their own family member, and most would want family present if they were the patient. Several themes emerged, including FPDR being a method to enhance staff and family communication, background of family members should determine permission to attend, and personal limitations of a nurse could be a barrier to FPDR. One obstacle identified was conflict between organizational and client/family culture, which could minimize the ability to accommodate individual beliefs. Comparatively, nurses with higher levels of nursing education and certified emergency nurses were more positive about FPDR.[13]

By contrast, a later study found no link between nurse education and support of FPDR.[14] Instead, investigators found a positive correlation between spirituality of nurses, physicians, and physician assistants (PAs) and support for FPDR, and found older HCPs tended to be less supportive of FPDR.[14]

Other researchers elucidated acute care nurses' beliefs about FPDR using interviews.[15] Analysis resulted in identification of 4 themes: conditions for FPDR, use of FPDR to force decision-making by family, staff's sense of being watched, and impact of FPDR on family. Diversity of responses led researchers to suggest an FP policy would reduce the influence of individual staff opinions, noting each resuscitation has variables to support or preclude the offer of FP.[15]

Research comparing perspectives of urban and suburban ED hospital personnel was conducted through a survey of physicians, nurses, PAs, and support staff in 4 Michigan hospitals.[16] Urbanites were less likely to support FPDR than HCPs in suburban settings. Opinions matched those relayed in other research, including concerns about distraction of HCPs, harmful psychological impact to family, problems of inadequate space, and fear of litigation.[16]

Elsewhere, a phenomenological approach was used to explore perceptions of acute care nurses who had experience with FPDR.[17] Four previously undescribed themes surfaced: the nurse forging a connection with family, engagement of family in care of the patient, nurses' transition to accept FPDR or IP, and the need for a cautious approach to FP. The experience could be exceptionally positive for the nurse, but some were ambivalent or held strong reservations about FP. The need to abide by legal and forensic rules in potential crimes was a barrier to allowing FP in certain cases.[17]

In 2008, a team of nurse researchers published 2 instruments related to FPDR: one to measure perceptions about risks and benefits to families, called the Family Presence Risk-Benefit Scale (FPR-BS), and another to measure self-confidence managing FPDR situations, called the Family Presence Self-Confidence Scale (FPS-CS).[18] The instruments were used initially in a study involving 375 RNs and LPNs. Survey scores were broadly distributed, reflecting divergent perspectives. Subjects who thought FPDR had more benefits and fewer risks indicated higher self-confidence managing FPDR. Nurses who belonged to professional organizations and those holding professional certifications had more positive scores on both scales, and ED nurses were more positive than nurses in other settings. Nurses with experience inviting FPDR perceived more benefits than risks and were more self-confident than those who did not.[18] This research introduced reliable, standardized instruments since used in other studies.[19,20]

Recently, the instruments were used to explore how different intensive care unit (ICU) environments affect nurses' perceptions of FPDR and IPs.[19] Nurses from the MICU and pediatric ICU (PICU) scored their confidence with managing FPDR situations and risk/benefit to the patient, family, and HCP higher than their counterparts in other ICUs, revealing differences between settings. Eighty-six percent of MICU nurses and 77% of PICU nurses had invited family to be present during resuscitation, whereas only 66% of surgical ICU nurses and 46% of nurses from other ICUs had done so.[19] These results reflect the importance of understanding baseline attitudes of staff about FPDR in unique clinical areas, because implementation tactics may depend on preexisting factors at the unit level.

International Health Care Provider Perspectives of Family Presence

HCPs, patients, and families in many countries may hail from diverse cultural backgrounds, bringing an international array of attitudes to the bedside. Because health practices have cultural variability, international studies offer insight into cultural aspects of FPDR.

In early FPDR research from Australia, investigators assessed ED staff members' attitudes about FPDR.[21] When asked if family should be invited to resuscitations, 62% would consider FPDR under controlled, predetermined circumstances, 14% indicated family should always be given the option, and 11% thought family should never be invited. Many (70%) favored the opportunity to attend their own relative's resuscitation.[21] This aspect illuminated a trend identified in other surveys[11,13]: HCPs themselves would like to receive the option of FPDR more often than those same HCPs support offering the option to patients' family members. Principal concerns were that the family may be disruptive or interfere, be offended by procedures or staff, or increase staff's emotional stress. Researchers concluded guidelines could help address the staff's apprehension.[21]

An Asian perspective was presented by examining attitudes held by ED staff in Singapore's largest hospital.[22] This study yielded some unique findings: only 14% of physicians and 3% of nurses thought relatives should be present during resuscitation, with no significant difference between professions. This finding departed from a pattern in other studies in which nurses were more supportive than physicians of FPDR.[11,12,21,23–26] Despite low HCP support for FPDR, approximately one-third of physicians and one-fourth of nurses indicated relatives had requested FPDR within the prior 6 months.[22] Of those who had experienced FPDR, 64.3% of physicians and 82.4% of nurses expressed discomfort with the situation. When asked to rate how relatives reacted to resuscitation, most selected descriptors were shock and disgust.[22] A study from Pakistan also revealed extremely low levels of HCP support, with 0% of physicians and 15% of nurses supporting FPDR.[27]

Nurse support has been low in other studies. In an investigation involving Turkish ICU nurses, 91.1% did not wish family to be present during CPR, and 88.9% thought doctors did not want family present.[28] Of 30 nurses who had experienced FPDR; two-thirds thought the experience had been negative. The researchers suggested education and guidelines may be helpful in enhancing experiences and practices.[28] Similarly, in an exploratory study of German ICU nurses' attitudes, more than two-thirds of respondents expressed disagreement with offering family the option to be present during resuscitation.[29] Of nurses who had been involved in FPDR, 65.7% indicated the experience was negative. Some subjects recounted instances of threats and physical violence toward the resuscitation team by family. Such experiences may cause reluctance to support FPDR. Despite negative experiences, some views were akin to those from other studies: FPDR should be individualized and situational; ideally, patient preferences should be gathered in advance; the need to support families; and family involvement in deciding when to terminate resuscitation.[29]

An exploration of European ICU nurses' attitudes revealed nurses in the United Kingdom tended to support FPDR more than their continental European counterparts.[30] Themes were similar to those found in United States research, including concerns about confidentiality and worries of families being upset by things said by the resuscitation team. Respondents mentioned having dedicated staff for family, but indicated staffing levels and space did not promote this. Most agreed family permitted to witness resuscitation would know all possible was being done, and 57.3% believed family should be allowed with the patient during the last moments of life. The investigators pointed out several factors that may have contributed to the array of responses, citing lack of experience, lack of solid evidence, traditions of paternalism, or practices of certain cultures.[30]

In a different cultural milieu, researchers sought the attitudes of nurses and physicians in Iranian hospitals, where FPDR generally is not practiced and the community is predominantly Muslim.[31] There, 77% of respondents opposed FPDR. ED physicians were more positive than nurses, general internists, and anesthesiologists. As identified elsewhere, the top concern about FPDR was psychological trauma for family. A unique recommendation was to provide public education about the possible benefits of FPDR.[31]

Voices of Patients and Families

HCPs have raised concerns about the impact on family from witnessing resuscitation of a loved one.[12,15–17,22,24,31] Logically, investigations of family members' responses to FPDR are necessary to assess the accuracy of HCPs' concerns. Fortunately, several studies have looked to family members, patients, and the public to gather perceptions, experiences, and beliefs.

Studies of health care provider, family, and patient views about family presence
Some investigators sought patient perspectives concomitantly with those of HCPs and families. For instance, attitudes about FPDR from family members who had witnessed IPs and resuscitation interventions, along with those of nurses and physicians, were explored following implementation of an FP guideline.[23] Of HCPs, nurses were most supportive of and comfortable with FP, followed closely by attending physicians. Residents lagged behind in terms of support and comfort, a trend also identified elsewhere.[23,25,26] Many positive effects were noted by family, negating staff concerns.[23] Staff, too, noted positive effects, including ensuring families knew everything possible had been done, staff being able to educate families, families being helpful to clinicians and the patient, and an enhanced sense of personhood of the patient. Concerns from staff included fear that prolonged resuscitation would occur, leading to worry about cost-benefit issues from increased staffing needs and treatment efforts.[23]

A study from the United Kingdom sought perspectives of HCPs along with those of patients with paired next of kin.[32] Most HCPs supported giving relatives the option of FPDR; support rose if the relative requested FPDR and was accompanied by trained staff. Half ranked the ability to explain resuscitation as the primary reason to allow FPDR and thought the greatest advantage was for relatives to see everything done for their family member. The principal reason for opposing FPDR was distress for family, an intriguing response because a significant number of these HCPs had participated in FPDR in an unstructured situation and, of those, most believed relatives had benefited and did not compromise the patient. Thoughts from patients and family members differed. Only 29% of patients desired FPDR, whereas 47% of relatives wished to attend. The main reason patients and relatives gave for FPDR was to provide support. Patients and families not wanting FPDR were concerned about family distress. Most thought their wishes should be documented, indicating they valued autonomy. The researchers proposed patients' wishes about FPDR should be honored if known.[32]

In another study capturing views of HCPs, patients, and family members, HCP respondents included 98 physicians, 98 nurses, and 6 respiratory therapists (RTs).[24] Overall, 54% of HCPs supported FPDR and IPs, and approximately two-thirds thought a policy was necessary. One HCP recommendation was to handle FPDR on a case-by-case basis depending on patient and family characteristics. Of family and patients surveyed, 31% and 29% had participated in FPDR or IPs, respectively. Family members who had experienced FP held more positive perspectives about being present, considered FP to be their right, wanted the option, and believed it was helpful to the patient. Almost all would participate in FP again. Patients echoed messages of family members: FP was their right, it would be comforting, and they should have the option.[24]

Family perspectives about family presence

Early research querying family members about FPDR came from the United Kingdom.[33] Thirty-five bereaved family members responded to a questionnaire inquiring whether they would have wished to be present in the ED during resuscitation efforts, and were asked to describe what they believed happens during resuscitation. Sixty-nine percent indicated they would have liked the option of FPDR, and 62% of those would have chosen to witness resuscitation. This finding illuminated the value they placed on being offered the option, even if they did not wish to attend. Beliefs about what happens during resuscitation ranged from somewhat accurate to nonsensical. The investigators concluded allowing families into the resuscitation may have benefits, as what they imagined might be worse than what really occurred, assurance may be provided that everything possible was being done.[33]

In the United States, researchers conducted a telephone survey of desires, beliefs, and concerns about FPDR with 25 family members of patients who had died in the ED of a large urban trauma center.[34] The majority thought FPDR should be offered, may have helped the patient, and would have helped their own grieving.[34] A study from another hospital in the United States described experiences of family members of patients who had survived CPR.[35] The major theme was family trying to decide whether to stay with the patient. Families wanted to know what was happening, and trusted HCPs to do their jobs caring for the patient. The investigators suggested that FPDR might meet families' needs for proximity to patients and information about patients' conditions.[35]

Family perspectives varied when investigators in Sweden explored family members' experiences and views about FPDR during a relative's resuscitation.[36] Resultant themes involved fear of disturbing resuscitation, whether the patient would desire their presence, what interviewees would want for themselves in such circumstances, whether family could cope, and whether FPDR added value. Most had neither attended nor been invited to the resuscitation, which they interpreted to mean that HCPs were against FPDR. A key point was the concept of FPDR as an option, allowing family the choice to decline or accept. The option is important because, as in an earlier study,[33] some people reported they definitely wanted to be there, whereas others definitely did not.[36]

Family preference for the option of FPDR also was found by investigators in Singapore after interviewing relatives of ED patients.[37] Family members were much more supportive of FPDR than medical staff in the same hospital had been in a prior study,[22] with 73.1% in favor compared with only 10.6% of the medical staff.[37] Subjects perceived FPDR would facilitate grieving, provide assurance everything possible had been done to save the patient, and create stronger bonds between family and medical staff. Relatives were less likely than medical staff to think FPDR would be traumatic for them or that their presence would cause stress to the resuscitation team.[37] The same mismatch was found in a study of predominantly Muslim bereaved family members in Pakistan.[27] HCPs were against FPDR, but 94% of family members indicated they wanted to be present during CPR and were not worried about what they would hear or see.[27]

The first randomized controlled trial (RCT) of FPDR examined psychological effects of witnessing resuscitation on relatives.[38] Relatives of ED patients were randomized to the experimental group, to whom the offer to attend resuscitation was made, or the control group, to whom no offer was made. A staff support person was present for all participants. Researchers halted the study early because of concerns that staff, who had concluded FPDR was beneficial, might threaten the experimental design. Despite study limitations, the results were interesting. Groups showed no differences in levels of distress. The experimental group showed a trend toward lower levels of grief symptoms, intrusive imagery, and posttraumatic avoidance than the control group. The researchers concluded beliefs FPDR would be psychologically harmful to family were unfounded. Three patients who survived resuscitation were asked about their comfort having family present; all felt supported and unconcerned with compromised dignity or confidentiality.[38]

Other investigators have explored the effect of FPDR on family members' depression and symptoms of posttraumatic stress disorder (PTSD). Comparing postbereavement depression and PTSD scores of family members who had witnessed resuscitation with those who had not, no significant differences in outcomes were found.[39]

Recently published results from a multicenter RCT focused on the effect of FPDR on PTSD symptoms in family, impact on medical efforts, well-being of HCPs, and medicolegal proceedings further support the benefits of FPDR and counter concerns of negative effects on the medical team.[40] Relatives in the intervention group were extended the option of attending resuscitation of their family member in the home; relatives in the control group were not. Subjects were interviewed 90 days after resuscitation. PTSD-related symptoms were significantly higher for those who had not witnessed resuscitation, as was incidence of anxiety. Those who had witnessed resuscitation had fewer symptoms of depression. Fewer than 1% of family members had conflict with the medical team or showed aggression. Twelve percent of those who had not witnessed CPR regretted not being there, whereas just 3% of those who had witnessed CPR expressed regrets of being present. FPDR had no impact on stress levels of medical teams, and there were no medicolegal conflicts.[40]

Patient perspectives
Patient preference is another aspect of FPDR. In one study exploring whether patients would want FPDR, most patients expressed a desire to have a family member present, although choice of family member varied.[41] Variation surfaced in another study when adults in an ED waiting room were asked if they would wish to attend a loved one's resuscitation, have a loved one attend their own resuscitation, or have a loved one attend their own resuscitation if that person wished to be present.[42] Regarding relatives attending their own resuscitation, the preference for a spouse to be present leaned toward the positive. For questions about most other relatives attending, responses hovered between uncertain and probably present. The majority tended not to want a minor child present. If a loved one wished to be present, responses for allowing FPDR were more favorable. Subjects were more likely to want to attend a relative's resuscitation than have a relative attend their own.[42]

Other research about patient views was conducted in 4 large hospitals in the United Kingdom.[43] Preferences about FPDR were collected from 61 adults, 21 of whom had been resuscitated. Overall, patients supported offering family the option and thought that family could provide support and advocate for the patient. Subjects indicated being present could provide family with acceptance of death, but some thought there may be times HCPs should use discretion if exposing family to unpleasant activities. Patients were not concerned about confidentiality, although sensitivity by HCPs discussing health information was desired, and a minority did not wish FPDR.[43]

Public perspectives

To gather public opinions outside of a health care setting, 408 adults in Pennsylvania were interviewed via telephone.[44] Compared with other surveys, respondents were more divisive about whether family members or friends should be allowed to witness resuscitation, with 49.3% agreeing or strongly agreeing, 22.4% being neutral, and 29.7% disagreeing or strongly disagreeing. Subjects also were asked if they would want to be present during a loved one's resuscitation, if they would want family or friends present during their own resuscitation, if FPDR would benefit the patient, and if it would benefit family and friends. Persons who would desire CPR themselves, those younger than 26 or older than 65 years, and those who were married, widowed, or never married expressed more positive responses toward FPDR. This study reiterated that many people want the option to be present or have loved ones present during resuscitation.[44] **Box 2** summarizes the opinions of patients, families, and the public.

INTERVENTIONS TO INFLUENCE HEALTH CARE PROVIDER ATTITUDES ABOUT FAMILY PRESENCE

Alongside uncovering HCP perspectives about FPDR, knowing how various factors influence attitudes can guide or change strategies. Several approaches have been tested, including education, policies, and practice guidelines.

Box 2
Thoughts about FPDR from family members, patients, and the public

Benefits

- It is a patient/family right
- Aids families' grieving
- Beneficial to patient; provides support and advocacy
- Less grief, intrusive imagery, and posttraumatic grief symptoms
- Families would know what was happening
- Family could be near the patient
- Questions could be answered
- Family would know all possible had been done
- Experience would strengthen bonds between medical team and family

Concerns

- Family distress from experience
- Family fear of disturbing resuscitation

General comments

- Patient preference to have family attend may vary by relationship to patient
- Would family add value to the resuscitation?
- Would patient want family present?
- HCPs should use discretion if exposing family to unpleasant activities and be sensitive when discussing health matters

Data from Refs.[9,17,23,24,27,32,34–38,40,41,43,44]

Education

One study examined whether a class about FPDR as a sole intervention could influence nurses' beliefs.[45] After attending class, nurses expressed greater support for offering the option. Nearly 80% indicated they planned to offer FPDR, compared with just 10.9% before the class.[45] Effects of education with additional interventions have also been explored. For instance, investigators surveyed ED nurses and physicians in a large urban hospital to assess changes in attitudes, behaviors, and values related to FPDR following education and guideline implementation.[26] After initial data collection, formal FPDR education was provided for nurses, whereas physicians received education during staff meetings. A guideline was developed, and offering FPDR began. Over time, FPDR was offered more frequently, often initiated by nurses who informed physicians about the practice. Remeasurement 1 year after implementation revealed 39% of nurses reported a more positive attitude about FPDR following education, with 36% expressing a more positive view after the FPDR program began, indicating both interventions may have helped shift nurse attitudes. Overall physician responses on the postintervention survey were, interestingly, less favorable toward FPDR and indicated more concerns about effects on resident education and legal issues, although caution was recommended in interpreting these results because of the small sample of physician respondents. The role of nurses as patient and family advocates in discussing benefits of FPDR with physician colleagues and the importance of reinforcing practice through ongoing education and dialogue were emphasized.[26]

Along similar lines, recent research measured the impact of HCP education about FPDR coupled with development of a unit-based guideline.[20] Postintervention data revealed more positive perceptions of FP risk-benefit, and more family members were invited to attend resuscitations, even though subjects did not rate themselves significantly more confident with FPDR. The proportion of HCPs who would want their own FPDR shifted from 39% to 58.5%. More than half (59%) thought FPDR should be the patient's decision, and 76% indicated this should be specified in an advance directive.[20]

Guidelines and Policies

Research suggests some HCPs favor policies or guidelines about FPDR.[21,24,25,30] Others have opposed such policies.[11] Still others have proposed that policies may not be necessary.[14] Key nursing organizations have addressed this topic, including the AACN, which advises having written policies, and ENA, which indicates a policy may aid in providing structure and support for HCPs.[4,6] How many organizations have formal policies or guidelines about FPDR is unknown at present, but has been assessed previously. More than a decade ago, published survey findings described policies, practices, and preferences of ICU and ED nurses related to FPDR and IPs.[46] Results reflected input from 984 RNs in the United States. Although only 5% of units had policies on FPDR, approximately half allowed FPDR in certain circumstances. More than one-third of respondents conveyed preference for written FPDR policies while slightly more did not favor policies. Even without policies, many nurses had taken family to the bedside during IPs or resuscitation, or would do so in the future.[46]

Subsequent research indicates policies are valued by HCPs. An interdisciplinary group harvested opinions of pediatric ED staff related to FPDR and IPs.[47] Overall, staff supported FPDR and IPs and desired an FP policy. Nurses were most supportive, followed by tenured medical staff. More novice resident physicians were less supportive of a policy.[47] The next year, after implementing FP, a second study at the same hospital evaluated how effectively the FP protocol facilitated uninterrupted care.[25] No instances of family interference with care occurred. Parents were overwhelmingly positive about the experience of FPDR, as were most HCPs. Nurses (92%) were more supportive of FPDR than attending physicians (78%). Only 35% of residents were supportive. Most HCPs believed FPDR was conditional on agreement of the physician in charge in addition to behavior and state of the parents, had no negative impact on patient care, and changed interpersonal dynamics of the health care team to a more professional communication level. A minority expressed concern that providing patient care was more difficult.[25]

Contemporary evidence suggests an FP protocol positively influences nurses' perceptions of benefits to family and increases nurses' confidence in their own contribution to resuscitation.[48] Nurses from an urban ED in which an FP protocol had been in place for more than 25 years held favorable views toward FPDR, and indicated other team members did also. FPDR occurred commonly, and no events were reported in which family experienced harm or took legal action. It was suggested long-term engagement in FPDR promotes acceptance by nurses and acceptance may be learned through modeling rather than a protocol.[48] These conclusions add strength to having a protocol, but emphasize the role of practicing FPDR in shaping nurses' perceptions.

The Impact of Experience

The aforementioned study and others show that experience with FPDR may contribute to positive HCP attitudes.[18,26,48] Research conducted in the pediatric realm revealed that nurses and attending physicians who had experienced FPDR were significantly more supportive than those without such experience.[49] Likewise, Duran and colleagues[24] found that HCPs who had been involved in FPDR held significantly more positive views than those who had not. In another study, physicians with more experience in practice and nurses with more experience with CPR, more experience with FPDR, and those who had received education about FPDR were more supportive of FPDR.[50] Further research may be helpful in ascertaining which interventions are most likely to enhance positive HCP attitudes about FPDR, and nurses interested in implementing the practice should consider what will work best in the context of their own professional environments.

THE AUTHORS' EXPERIENCE WITH FAMILY PRESENCE DURING RESUSCITATION

In 2011, a project to change practice around FPDR was initiated in the 24-bed MICU of a large, urban, tertiary-care, academic medical center. At the time there was no standard of practice in the hospital or in the MICU allowing FPDR, and it occurred very rarely.

The project began with a survey administered to MICU nurses and hospital chaplains to gather baseline attitudes and beliefs toward the subject. Assessing staff members' knowledge and comfort with FP, patient-/family-centered care, and aspects regarding psycho-social-spiritual support is valuable when beginning an FP initiative.[51] Chaplains were included because a chaplain attends every resuscitation attempt, often to support and communicate with family members; therefore, involving and educating chaplains about the practice change was important for success. Although physicians were not surveyed, the MICU medical director and other key critical care physicians were informed about project plans and support moving forward.

One presurvey question asked respondents to share personal concerns regarding FP. Some individuals were very concerned about implementing FP, with several remarks parallel to those found in the literature. One person wrote "please don't implement this" on the survey. Although nurses and chaplains voiced apprehension, comments supporting the implementation of FP were also offered. Specific staff responses are listed in **Box 3**. Survey feedback was used to help develop content and plan staff education by ensuring issues raised by staff could be addressed with evidence-based information.

A review of current literature about FPDR was used to formulate education materials, including a pamphlet summarizing reasons family members desire to be present, staff fears about FP, and facts about FP. A PowerPoint presentation available on the AACN Web site was also used for education.[52] Education was provided face-to-face by the nurse leading the project.

Following education, staff completed a 2-question survey: (1) List 2 benefits of FPDR you learned about; and (2) What was the most valuable part of the presentation? Answers to the first question included: FPDR helps bring closure for family; families see everything was done; it reduces fears; there is no evidence of problems with FPDR; and it allows families to share last moments with loved ones. Responses to the second question included: learning how beneficial FP can be with no negative outcomes; knowing most families would like the option to be present; learning research had been done was a motivator to implement evidence-based practice around FPDR; and education dispelled myths. After this, attitudes of staff toward FP shifted toward a more inclusive practice. It was no longer their first instinct to ask family to leave if resuscitation became necessary. Not long after FP education occurred, a hospital policy promoting patient and family-centered care was implemented, permitting patients and families to be together in the MICU most of the time. This concomitant change from more restricted visitation helped advance staff acceptance of FP during patient

---

Box 3
Baseline feedback from MICU nurses and hospital chaplains about FPDR

Benefits

- "Especially during CPR family should be offered the chance to be in the room. It is the most important policy we could have"

- "It could be beneficial to humanize the patient for the team, comfort for the patient when conscious, understanding of CPR for the family, and sense of helping by being present"

- "Family can have a more realistic view of what their sick family member has to endure during CPR"

Concerns

- Fear of making a mistake

- "This is a violent event and perhaps not suited for all"

- Potential distractions/interference by emotional outbursts, misconception/misunderstanding of code team humor, potential effects of family exposure to the trauma of CPR, intubation, and so forth"

- "I do not want distraction. The patient and their safety have got to be the primary focus"

- "May create anxiety and increase pressure/stress to the medical team, especially when it's a team of medical residents who are building up their skills"

General comments

- "Depends on the situation, it could show family we did all we could do and help with their coping"

care activities, including resuscitation. A case study describing an FPDR experience is presented in **Box 4**.

FPDR is now strongly supported in the MICU. During resuscitation events nurses ask, "Is there any family? Do we need to get them?" Expected practice is to bring family to the bedside as quickly as possible if they are not already in the room. One nurse, who initially adamantly opposed FPDR, became a supporter after witnessing the benefit it had on her patient's family and their ability to cope. Newly hired nurses learn about FPDR during orientation to acquaint them with unit expectations. A future goal is to spread FPDR across the hospital with a standardized guideline for the practice.

DISCUSSION

Despite decades of research, inconsistencies remain around FPDR, largely hinging on divergent attitudes of HCPs. Ongoing beliefs that FPDR is harmful to families and patients are unsubstantiated by research; rather, synthesis of available data indicates actual and perceived benefits outweigh the risks. Nurses wishing to implement FPDR should consider several points:

- Before implementing an FPDR program, assess the environment including current HCP beliefs about FPDR, interprofessional dynamics, leadership support for change, and available resources to initiate and sustain the practice.
- Education about FPDR has been effective in positively shifting HCP attitudes about FPDR. Those in teaching hospitals should include resident physicians. Because resuscitation involves several disciplines, an interdisciplinary approach is advised.
- Beliefs about FPDR vary by culture; therefore, understanding cultural preferences of patients, families, and other HCPs is as valuable in FPDR as in other patient care issues.

Box 4
Case study

Late one evening, nurses in the MICU heard a page announcing a code on the oncology unit just down the hall. Nurses from the MICU went to help because they knew they could get there quickly to initiate ACLS. As they got to the room, oncology nurses were performing chest compressions on Mrs S., a 70-year-old woman with a history of ovarian cancer who had become unresponsive and pulseless. Mrs S.'s sister was standing in the corner of the room trying to stay out of the way. The code team arrived shortly after the ICU nurses and Mrs S. regained a pulse after 10 minutes of ACLS. Mrs S. was intubated and then the code team transported her to the MICU. Mrs S.'s sister, who had remained present throughout the code, went with them. She had called Mrs S.'s husband to let him know what was going on. He had gone home but was heading back to hospital after learning of the situation. On arrival to the MICU, Mrs S. was hooked up to the ICU monitor and her vital signs were reassessed. She was hypotensive and bradycardic. Shortly thereafter she lost her pulse again. The entire code team was still present, and chest compressions and ACLS interventions resumed. Unfortunately, despite ongoing efforts, Mrs S. did not recover and resuscitation efforts were terminated. The MICU nurses had been educated about the importance of FPDR, so had allowed Mrs S.'s sister to remain in the room with her. The sister was able to say goodbye to Mrs S. and witness the efforts of the code team. Mr S. arrived 20 minutes after resuscitation efforts ceased. He was very upset, angry, and could not understand how this had happened. He wanted an explanation, because when he had been with Mrs S. earlier, everything had seemed fine. Because Mrs S.'s sister had witnessed everything, she explained to him how hard everyone had worked to try and save his wife's life. She was able to comfort him with the fact that she had been there, and his wife was not alone.

- Ideally, individual patient preferences about FPDR should be ascertained and documented before a resuscitation event.
- Having a designated family support a person during resuscitation events is likely to benefit family and allow staff to focus on the patient.
- A policy or guideline for FPDR may help support practice change and consistency.
- In general, HCPs with more FPDR experience are more supportive of the practice. Consider leveraging this by having experienced HCPs share positive experiences.
- Exceptions to offering FPDR should be consistent, and may include legal restrictions or situations when relatives pose a threat to the patient or HCPs.

SUMMARY

Whenever possible, patient care, including practices around FPDR, should be based on evidence. Current variations in practice lead to inequities in care. It is unethical to offer the option of FPDR to some individuals and not to others based on the subjective views of the resuscitation team when there is substantial evidence to support the practice. Nurses can positively influence patients, families, and the health care team by advocating for or leading a thoughtful, consistent, evidence-based approach to FPDR.

REFERENCES

1. Berg RA, Hemphill R, Abella BS, et al. Part 5: adult basic life support: 2010 American Heart Association guidelines for cardiopulmonary resuscitation and emergency cardiovascular care. Circulation 2010;122(18):S685–705. http://dx.doi.org/10.1161/CIRCULATIONAHA.110.970939. Accessed December 2, 2013.
2. Neumar RW, Otto CW, Link MS, et al. Part 8: adult advanced cardiovascular life support: 2010 American Heart Association guidelines for cardiopulmonary resuscitation and emergency cardiovascular care. Circulation 2010;122(18):S729–67. http://dx.doi.org/10.1161/CIRCULATIONAHA.110.970988. Accessed December 2, 2013.
3. Morrison LJ, Kierzek G, Diekema DS, et al. Part 3: ethics: 2010 American Heart Association guidelines for cardiopulmonary resuscitation and emergency cardiovascular care. Circulation 2010;122(18):S665–75. http://dx.doi.org/10.1161/CIRCULATIONAHA.110.970905.
4. American Association of Critical Care Nurses. AACN practice alert: family presence during resuscitation and invasive procedures. 2010. Available at: http://www.aacn.org/wd/practice/docs/practicealerts/family%20presence%2004-2010%20final.pdf. Accessed December 2, 2013.
5. Davidson JE, Powers K, Hedayat KM, et al. Clinical practice guidelines for support of the family in the patient-centered intensive care unit: American College of Critical Care Medicine Task Force 2004–2005. Crit Care Med 2007;35(2):605–22. Available at: http://www.learnicu.org/docs/guidelines/patient-centeredintensive.pdf. Accessed December 2, 2013.
6. Wolf L, Storer A, Barnason S, et al. Emergency Nurses Association clinical practice guideline: family presence during invasive procedures and resuscitation. 2012. Available at: http://www.ena.org/practice-research/research/CPG/Documents/FamilyPresenceCPG.pdf. Accessed December 2, 2013.
7. Henderson DP, Knapp JF. Report of the national consensus conference on family presence during pediatric cardiopulmonary resuscitation and procedures. Pediatr Emerg Care 2005;21(11):787–91.

8. The Joint Commission. R3 Report. 2011. Available at: http://www.joint commission.org/assets/1/18/r3%20report%20issue%201%2020111.pdf. Accessed December 2, 2013.

9. Doyle CJ, Post H, Burney RE, et al. Family participation during resuscitation: an option. Ann Emerg Med 1987;16(6):673–5.

10. Hanson C, Strawser D. Family presence during cardiopulmonary resuscitation: Foote Hospital emergency department's nine-year perspective. J Emerg Nurs 1992;18(2):104–6.

11. Helmer SD, Smith S, Dort JM, et al. Family presence during trauma resuscitation: a survey of AAST and ENA members. J Trauma 2000;48(6):1015–24.

12. McClenathan BM, Torrington KG, Uyehara CF. Family member presence during cardiopulmonary resuscitation: a survey of US and international critical care professionals. Chest 2002;122(6):2204–11.

13. Ellison S. Nurses' attitudes toward family presence during resuscitative efforts and invasive procedures. J Emerg Nurs 2003;29(6):515–21.

14. Baumhover N, Hughes L. Spirituality and support for family presence during resuscitations in adults. Am J Crit Care 2009;18(4):357–66. http://dx.doi.org/10.4037/ajcc2009759.

15. Knott A, Kee CC. Nurses' beliefs about family presence during resuscitation. Appl Nurs Res 2005;18(4):192–8.

16. Macy C, Lampe E, O'Neil B, et al. The relationship between the hospital setting and perceptions of family-witnessed resuscitation in the emergency department. Resuscitation 2006;70(1):74–9. http://dx.doi.org/10.1016/j.resuscitation.2005.11.013.

17. Miller JH, Stiles A. Family presence during resuscitation and invasive procedures: the nurse experience. Qual Health Res 2009;19(10):1431–42. http://dx.doi.org/10.1177/1049732309348365.

18. Twibell RS, Siela D, Riwitis C, et al. Nurses' perceptions of their self-confidence and the benefits and risks of family presence during resuscitation. Am J Crit Care 2008;17:101–12.

19. Carroll DL. The effect of intensive care unit environments on nurse perceptions of family presence during resuscitation and invasive procedures. Dimens Crit Care Nurs 2014;33(1):34–9. http://dx.doi.org/10.1097/DCC.0000000000000010.

20. Edwards EE, Despotopulos LD, Carroll DL. Changes in provider perceptions of family presence during resuscitation. Clin Nurse Spec 2013;27(5):239–44. http://dx.doi.org/10.1097/NUR.0b013e3182a0ba13.

21. Redley B, Hood K. Staff attitudes towards family presence during resuscitation. Accid Emerg Nurs 1996;4(3):145–51.

22. Ong ME, Chan YH, Srither DE, et al. Asian medical staff attitudes towards witnessed resuscitation. Resuscitation 2004;60(1):45–50.

23. Meyers TA, Eichhorn DJ, Guzzetta CE, et al. Family presence during invasive procedures and resuscitation: the experience of family members, nurses and physicians. Am J Nurs 2000;100(2):32–43.

24. Duran CR, Oman KS, Abel JJ, et al. Attitudes toward and beliefs about family presence: a survey of healthcare providers, patients' families, and patient. Am J Crit Care 2007;16(3):270–9.

25. Mangurten JA, Scott SH, Guzzetta CE, et al. Effects of family presence during resuscitation and invasive procedures in a pediatric emergency department. J Emerg Nurs 2006;32(3):225–33.

26. Mian P, Warchal S, Whitney S, et al. Impact of a multifaceted intervention on nurses' and physicians' attitudes and behaviors toward family presence during resuscitation. Crit Care Nurse 2007;27(1):52–61.

27. Zakaria M, Siddique M. Presence of family members during cardio-pulmonary resuscitation after necessary amendments. J Pak Med Assoc 2008;58(11):632–5.
28. Gunes UY, Zaybek A. A study of Turkish critical care nurses' perspectives regarding family-witnessed resuscitation. J Clin Nurs 2009;18(20):2907–15. http://dx.doi.org/10.1111/j.1365-2702.2009.02826.x.
29. Koberich S, Kaltwasser A, Rothaug O, et al. Family witnessed resuscitation-experience and attitudes of German intensive care nurses. Nurs Crit Care 2010;15(5):241–50. http://dx.doi.org/10.1111/j.1478-5153.2010.00405.x.
30. Fulbrook P, Albarran JW, Latour JM. European survey of critical care nurses' attitudes and experiences of having family members present during cardiopulmonary resuscitation. Int J Nurs Stud 2005;42(5):557–68.
31. Kianmehr N, Mofidi M, Rahmani H, et al. The attitudes of team members towards family presence during hospital-based CPR: a study based in the Muslim setting of four Iranian teaching hospitals. J R Coll Physicians Edinb 2010;40(1):4–8. http://dx.doi.org/10.4997/JRCPE.2010.102.
32. Grice AS, Picton P, Deakin CD. Study examining attitudes of staff, patients and relatives to witnessed resuscitation in adult intensive care units. Br J Anaesth 2003;91(6):820–4.
33. Barratt F, Wallis DN. Relatives in the resuscitation room: their point of view. J Accid Emerg Med 1998;15(2):109–11.
34. Meyers TA, Eichhorn DJ, Guzzetta CE. Do family members want to be present during CPR? A retrospective survey. J Emerg Nurs 1998;24(5):400–5.
35. Wagner JM. Lived experience of critically ill patients' family members during cardiopulmonary resuscitation. Am J Crit Care 2004;13(5):416–20.
36. Weslien M, Nilstun T, Lundquist A, et al. Narratives about resuscitation – family members differ about presence. Eur J Cardiovasc Nurs 2006;5(1):68–74.
37. Ong ME, Chung WL, Mei JS. Comparing attitudes of the public and medical staff towards witnessed resuscitation in an Asian population. Resuscitation 2007;73(1):103–5.
38. Robinson SM, Mackenzie-Ross S, Hewson GL, et al. Psychological effect of witnessed resuscitation on bereaved relatives. Lancet 1998;352(9128):614–7.
39. Compton S, Levy P, Griffin M, et al. Family witnessed resuscitation: bereavement outcomes in an urban environment. J Palliat Med 2011;14(6):715–21. http://dx.doi.org/10.1089/jpm.2010.0463.
40. Jabre P, Belpomme V, Azoulay E, et al. Family presence during cardiopulmonary resuscitation. N Engl J Med 2013;368(11):1008–18. http://dx.doi.org/10.1056/NEJMoa1203366.
41. Benjamin M, Holger J, Carr M. Personal preferences regarding family member presence during resuscitation. Acad Emerg Med 2004;11(7):750–3.
42. Berger JT, Brody G, Eisenstein L, et al. Do potential recipients of cardiopulmonary resuscitation want their family members to attend? A survey of public preferences. J Clin Ethics 2004;15(3):237–42.
43. Mcmahon-Parkes K, Moule P, Benger J, et al. The views and preferences of resuscitated and non-resuscitated patients towards family-witnessed resuscitation: a qualitative study. Int J Nurs Stud 2009;46(2):220–9. http://dx.doi.org/10.1016/j.ijnurstu.2008.08.007.
44. Mazer MA, Cox LA, Capon JA. The public's attitude and perception concerning witnessed cardiopulmonary resuscitation. Crit Care Med 2006;34(12):2925–8. http://dx.doi.org/10.1097/01.CCM.0000247720.99299.77.
45. Bassler PC. The impact of education on nurses' beliefs regarding family presence in a resuscitation room. J Nurses Staff Dev 1999;15(3):126–31.

46. MacLean SL, Guzzetta CE, White C, et al. Family presence during cardiopulmonary resuscitation and invasive procedures: practices of critical care and emergency nurses. Am J Crit Care 2003;12(23):246–57.
47. Mangurten JA, Scott SH, Guzzetta CE, et al. Family presence: making room. Am J Nurs 2005;105(5):40–8.
48. Lowry E. "It's just what we do": a qualitative study of emergency nurses working with well-established family presence protocol. J Emerg Nurs 2012;38(4): 329–34. http://dx.doi.org/10.1016/j.jen.2010.12.016.
49. Sacchetti A, Carraccio C, Leva E, et al. Acceptance of family member presence during pediatric resuscitation in the emergency department: effects of personal experience. Pediatr Emerg Care 2000;16(2):85–7.
50. Feagan LM, Fisher NJ. The impact of education on provider attitudes toward family-witnessed resuscitation. J Emerg Nurs 2011;37(3):231–9. http://dx.doi.org/10.1016/j.jen.2010.02.023.
51. Emergency Nurses Association. Presenting the option for family presence. 3rd edition. Des Plaines (IL): Emergency Nurses Association; 2007.
52. American Association of Critical Care Nurses. Family presence during resuscitation and invasive procedures. Family Presence Presentation. PPT: - 4/2010. Available at: http://www.aacn.org/wd/practice/content/family-presence-practice-alert.pcms?menu=practice. Accessed December 2, 2013.

Palliative Care in the Intensive Care Unit

Jame Restau, MSN, RN, ACNS-BC, ACHPN[a],*, Pamela Green, MSN, RN, FNP-BC[b]

KEYWORDS

- Palliative care • Intensive care • Quality • Patient- and family-centered care
- Complex adaptive system

KEY POINTS

- High-quality care for intensive care patients and their families should include palliative care.
- Nearly half of all patients who die in the hospital receive intensive care services during their terminal admission.
- One of the key goals of health care is to limit costs while simultaneously improving or maintaining the quality of care that patients and families receive.
- Quality measures for palliative care in the ICU are being developed at a national level and can be implemented in diverse ICUs across the nation.

Restorative care and comfort care are often seen as mutually exclusive. Promulgating this misconception are insurance mandates that patients forgo curative treatment when seeking comfort and symptom management in the face of terminal illness. This dichotomy of care has created barriers to early access of palliative services for the patient and their families. Providing quality of care to patients with life-limiting illness is the challenge facing the staff in the intensive care unit (ICU).

IMPORTANCE OF THE PROBLEM

Although the Bible reminds us that "there is a time to be born and a time to die," we have paid strikingly little attention to the "time to die" until recently. In ancient times, death was quick and often sudden. Now death most often occurs during the course of prolonged chronic illness that may last years. Patients may experience serious physical, emotional, social, and spiritual suffering. In addition, such patients, their families, the physicians and nurses, and others involved in the delivery of care face ethical

Disclosure Statement: J. Restau nor P. Green have any disclosures to claim.
[a] Department of Supportive and Palliative Care, Baylor Medical Center at Irving, 1901 North MacArthur Boulevard, Irving, TX 75061, USA; [b] Department of Supportive and Palliative Care, Baylor Regional Medical Center at Carrollton, 4343 N. Josey Lane, Carrollton, TX 75010, USA
* Corresponding author.
E-mail address: Jame.Restau@baylorhealth.edu

Crit Care Nurs Clin N Am 26 (2014) 551–558
http://dx.doi.org/10.1016/j.ccell.2014.08.013
0899-5885/14/$ – see front matter © 2014 Elsevier Inc. All rights reserved.
ccnursing.theclinics.com

and financial challenges.[1] Curative and palliative care should be provided congruently to meet the needs of all partners in a patient's care. The symptom burden of disease, communication of goals of care, alignment of treatment and therapy to goals, values and preferences, and appropriate, timely transition of care should not be limited by prognosis.[2]

REVIEW OF THE LITERATURE

The United States has seen a decline in the number of hospitals since early 1986; however, some areas report up to a 26% increase in the number of intensive care beds. Occupancy rates and average length of stay in the ICUs are increasing.[3] One in five patients receives terminal care in the intensive care setting.[4] Approximately 90% of deaths in the ICU occur after discontinuing or limiting treatment.[5] Of all hospital deaths, 47% receive intensive care services during the terminal admission[6] with less than 20% of these patients having completed an advance directive.[7] Do-not-attempt-resuscitation orders are often written within days of death. Because these conversations occur late in the disease trajectory, patients and families perceive this dialogue as a sign of impending doom rather than a result of advance care planning.[8]

Family members making decisions for their loved ones often continue treatment despite prior conversations with the patient to the contrary.[9] These decisions create emotional distress and financial burden on the family.[10] In turn, the decisions made or not made by the family can cause moral distress for the caregivers as continuing aggressive care becomes more burdensome than beneficial for the patient. Poor understanding of diagnosis, prognosis, and treatment options has been identified in 54% of family members with loved ones suffering serious illness. Families have the perception that health care providers experience stress when discussing end of life in the ICU,[5] which can often lead to families second-guessing themselves in regards to the care decisions they have made.

It is well documented that the last chapter of life is characterized by three major deficiencies: (1) unnecessary suffering,[11] (2) unacceptable variation in treatment with striking excesses in nonbeneficial treatment,[12] and (3) unsustainable costs. Approximately 30% of Centers of Medicare and Medicaid Services dollars have been attributed to end-of-life care.[13] A total of 40% of Centers of Medicare and Medicaid Services costs occur in the last 30 days of life.[14] The number of Americans age 65 and older will double by 2030.[3] Too many patients get too much medical intervention, too little advance care planning, and too little care in the last chapter of life.

In response to these deficits, the National Consensus Project for Quality Palliative Care and the National Quality Forms established standards for high-quality palliative care. The Institute of Medicine, the major societies representing critical care health care professionals, government and industry health care payers, along with large-scale health care systems across the nation agree that palliative care in the ICU should be a quality improvement priority.[10] The Center to Advance Palliative Care developed an ICU-focused initiative (Improving Palliative Care in the Intensive Care Unit) in 2010 where health care systems could assess resources, guidelines, and expertise. These recommendations have been used to guide the development of ICU palliative care programs and establish standards for tracking and benchmarking for quality. A consensus of expert professional opinion developed domains for quality palliative care (**Box 1**). Integrating these features into the ICU can be difficult because each has its own culture created by history, structures of care, policies and procedures, and the attitudes and professional interaction between the different disciplines working in the critical care setting.[15]

Box 1
Professionals' definition of domains of ICU palliative care quality from the Robert Wood Johnson Foundation Critical Care End-of-Life Peer Workgroup
Symptoms management and comfort care
Communication within team and with patients and families
Patient- and family-centered decision making
Emotional and practical support for patients and families
Spiritual support for patients and families
Continuity of care
Emotional and organizational support for ICU clinicians
Data from Clarke EB, Curtis JR, Luce JM, et al. Quality indicators for end-of-life care in the intensive care unit. Crit Care Med 2003;31:2255–62.

Poor-quality end-of-life care creates stress for the patient, family, and health care providers. Lack of and/or limited access to palliative care can result in higher costs and more aggressive care at the end of life. Family members suffer posttraumatic stress disorder and extended grieving with prolongation of the death process in their loved ones. Nelson and colleagues[16] stress the importance family members place on early attempts to elicit the patient's values and treatment preferences, because this decreases the burden and guilt family members feel when making treatment decisions for their loved one. Health care providers witness patient and family suffering, high mortality, inappropriate care, and poor resource stewardship, which lead to intensive care staff burnout.[17]

As part of a large health care system in Northeast Texas committed to patient-centered care, supportive and palliative care programs have been established in half of the acute care facilities throughout the health care system. As part of this initiative, significant gains have been realized in the quality of care delivered in the ICUs. Interdisciplinary critical care teams help to identify those patients who would likely benefit from supportive and palliative care services.

Screening criteria has been implemented across the health care system. This screening process has been implemented in the ICUs and on admission in some facilities. Palliative care consultation is included on ventilator order sets with a prompt for palliative care screen on ventilator Day 4. The emergency departments are also initiating a screening tool to identify patients appropriate for palliative care services earlier to decrease the number of readmissions. A standardized order set has been developed for withdrawal of mechanical ventilation. By establishing standardized protocols, clinicians are provided practice recommendations to ensure patient comfort during the withdrawal process.

For the first quarter of fiscal year 2014, of those patients admitted, 3.6% to 5.0% received a palliative care consultation (**Fig. 1**). The percentage of palliative care consultations originating in the ICU ranged from 26.5% to 45% (**Fig. 2**). *Hospital A* is the largest hospital in the health care system and also the site of the first palliative care program within the system. *Hospital B* is a community hospital where the first palliative care advanced practice registered nurse was hired in 2008. *Hospital C* is a new program that began in 2010. The final percentage, *Hospital D*, represents the percentage of consultations as a whole from all palliative care programs within the health care system. Palliative care was consulted in 4.8% of the patients admitted to medical and surgical services. On average, 26.5% of all palliative care consultations originated in the

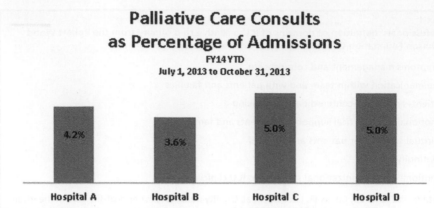

Fig. 1. Palliative care consultations as percentage of admission.

ICU. Patients seen by palliative care made different decisions regarding resuscitation status with 49% choosing do-not-attempt-resuscitation status.

CASE STUDIES

Two case studies are provided to demonstrate the benefit of supportive and palliative care services in providing patient- and family-centered care. Nursing and medical staff benefit in time saved and emotional support is also realized. These case studies highlight opportunity for improvement.

Case #1

AG presented to his primary care provider with increasing cough, dyspnea, and associated elevated temperature worsening over the previous 48 hours. He had a history of chronic obstructive pulmonary disease, having smoked cigarettes for 50 years. He quit smoking 15 years ago. He also had a history of osteoarthritis and hearing loss "since the military." He lived alone in a single-story house. He had been widowed for 10 years, his wife dying of cancer. He volunteered at his church and assisted other members with transportation needs and errands.

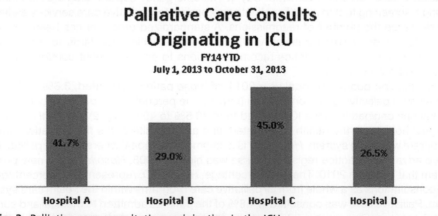

Fig. 2. Palliative care consultations originating in the ICU.

AG had not completed an advanced directive despite conversations with his primary care provider and his family members. AG believed his children would "do the right thing if something happened."

AG was admitted to the hospital with community-acquired pneumonia complicated by chronic obstructive pulmonary disease. Intravenous antibiotics, steroids, nebulizer treatments, and oxygen therapy were initiated. Despite treatment, his condition deteriorated requiring intensive care. Because of loss of decision-making capacity, AG's children were approached to make decisions regarding their father's treatment. The children expressed their concern that their father would never want to be "kept alive by machines." The intensivist believed the patient had a good change for recovery, but sensed hesitancy from the family to proceed with ventilator support. The intensivist consulted the supportive and palliative care team for goal setting and treatment options.

The palliative care advanced practice registered nurse and physician met with the family. Prognosis and likelihood for meaningful recovery were discussed. The family was educated on the disease trajectory of chronic obstructive pulmonary disease. Through reflection and storytelling, the family was able to come to a definition for quality of life that would be acceptable for their father. The children made a decision for a limited trial of ventilator support to afford their father an opportunity to improve.

Despite maximum treatment and ventilator support, AG's condition continued to decline. The family was able to make a decision for withdrawal of treatment, allowing their father to pass peacefully. Although difficult, the decision to withdraw treatment was made with the knowledge that every opportunity for recovery had been afforded the patient. The family was confident they had represented their father's wishes.

Case #2

DD is a 22-year-old man diagnosed with acute lymphoblastic leukemia at age 5. The patient had been in complete remission after a bone marrow transplant at age 9. Since that time, he has been active, graduated from high school, and was currently in his senior year of college.

DD presented to the hospital with intense right lower extremity pain, onset 1 week before arrival. The pain was attributed to possible injury when helping a friend move. A radiograph was performed by his primary care provider and found to be abnormal. The patient was admitted to the hospital for further diagnostic evaluation.

Diagnostic testing revealed an elevated white count and decreased platelets. Magnetic resonance imaging showed increased uptake in the right femur, pelvis, and perihilar lymph nodes. Bone biopsy revealed leukemia. Treatment was initiated within 48 hours of diagnosis.

The patient tolerated the initial cycle of chemotherapy well; however, he developed neutropenia. He later became septic and was placed on appropriate antibiotic therapy. His condition deteriorated requiring transfer to the ICU, where he was placed on vasopressors. The patient and family chose to continue aggressive treatment despite the deterioration in overall condition, the presence of elevated temperature, and the need for continuous renal-replacement therapy.

The patient's condition deteriorated requiring endotracheal intubation and ventilation. The health care team met with the family to discuss overall prognosis and reasonable expectations for a meaningful recovery. The family believed "the physicians weren't trying hard enough." The meeting ended with the family insisting "everything continue to be done." The health care team felt frustrated and confused about the family's expectations.

After several more days of continued aggressive treatment with no improvement in overall condition, the family asked to have the patient transferred to another facility. The patient's family had retained legal counsel and the health care providers felt pressure to comply with the family request, despite their belief the patient was not stable for transfer. Amid objection from various members of the health care team, an accepting physician and receiving facility were secured and emergency medical transport was arranged to provide transfer. The patient suffered a cardiac arrest en route to the accepting facility. Resuscitative measures were unsuccessful. The family was angry, blaming the health care team for not providing adequate care. The health care team believed they had failed the patient by facilitating the transfer.

These case studies show how the components of palliative care can affect the outcomes for patients and families in the critical care setting. AG's case study demonstrates how a palliative care team can improve the communication between care providers and families by assisting with difficult conversation, identifying and addressing goals of care, and providing quality end-of-life care within a critical care setting. These principles can be adopted by any critical care team and unit with or without a palliative care team in place. DD's story occurs far too often in critical care units across the nation. By including palliative care, many of the stressors experienced by the patient, family, and care providers could have been decreased or eliminated. Palliative care would have helped address the patient's and parents concerns about aggressive interventions and assisted in the understanding and ultimate acceptance of his prognosis by managing expectation through the use of family meetings, clarification of goals of care, and symptom management.

RELATION TO THE COMPLEX ADAPTIVE SYSTEM

The study of complex adaptive science or systems developed from the roots of biology, physics, and mathematics and has expanded to organizations, such as health care systems.[18] Health care systems are a prime example of a complex adaptive system because of the diversity of systems and the complexity of interactions and interdependence. There are four common features of complex adaptive systems: (1) dynamic states, (2) massive entanglement, (4) emergent, and (4) robust.[18]

Health care systems are influenced by connections and forces to make changes. Connections are internal and external to the practice environment. The ICU is constantly undergoing changes because of such factors as staffing, practice guidelines, and advances in technology. Evidence-based practice has been one of the strongest external forces for change in health care. Evidence-based practice supports the integration of palliative care into the ICU to improve quality of care for patients and families approaching end of life. The relationships within an ICU can make integration of palliative care difficult. Physicians and other health care providers may be hesitant to use palliative care services because of lack of exposure or education about the services that palliative care can provide for patients, families, and staff. Physicians and nurses have a complex and interdependent relationship in an ICU. One cannot function without the support, engagement, and skill of the other. They adapt to each other's behaviors in regards to the intensity and focus of patient care. This interdependence can be a positive and negative factor for palliative care. If either factor has negative feelings or prior experience with palliative care, it can block the ability for palliative care to provide patient- and family-centered care. Yet, these same forces can be used to create change in the ICU one patient experience at a time.

Small changes to bedside care and communication can lead to large changes in the ICU. These small changes can spread quickly throughout a complex adaptive system to change the exact path that it follows in the future. The same relationship within families can change the care in an ICU. The relationship between and among family members can lead to tension and stress for the physicians and nurses. These relationships can further complicate the care of the patient because differences in opinion can lead to prolonged suffering for the patient, family, and staff at the bedside. The robustness or fitness of the ICU is altered based on feedback, the type of feedback received from physicians, patients, and families. Feedback can come in the form of surveys, letters, and face-to-face communication between physicians, families, and staff. This communication can help validate the role of palliative care in an ICU.

IMPLICATIONS FOR PRACTICE

Major stakeholders are calling for changes in health care with regard to focus and intensity of care at the end of life. A key goal of health care is to limit costs while simultaneously improving or maintaining the quality of care that patients and families receive. One way to achieve this goal is through integration of palliative care in the ICU for patients suffering from terminal and/or life-limiting illness, providing comfort, care, and planning to achieve their personal goals.

The ICU environment can be overwhelming, scary, and confusing for patients and families. One of the major stressors of an ICU is the uncertainty that often accompanies the patient with a terminal and/or chronic condition. Palliative care offers a service to patients and families that can help to alleviate some of the stress and uncertainty during an ICU admission. This support, communication, and coordination improve the quality of care received by the patient and family while assisting the medical staff by decreasing the burden of care.

Integrating palliative care into the ICU improves outcomes for patients and families. Palliative care helps to direct the focus of care and ensures that every patient admitted to the ICU has his or her dignity maintained through supportive, encouraging, and compassionate communication. Palliative care clinicians can work with intensive care clinicians to provide families with timely, clear, and compassionate communication about their loved one's prognosis. Medical decision making should be aligned with the patient's values, goals, and treatment preferences either through the use of advance directives or shared decision making by the family, which can be determined through family meetings. Families and significant others should be offered interdisciplinary support from such services as palliative care, chaplains, social work, and care coordination to improve quality outcomes. By bringing these simple principles to the bedside, the ICU improves outcomes for patients, families, physicians, and staff.

REFERENCES

1. Nelson JE, Cortez TB, Curtis JR, et al. Integrating palliative care in the ICU. J Hosp Palliat Nurs 2011;13:89–94. http://dx.doi.org/10.1097/NJH.0b013e318203d9ff.
2. Nelson JE, Campbell ML, Curtis JR, et al. Defining standards for ICU palliative care: a brief review from the IPAL-ICU project. Center to Advance Palliative Care. 2010. Available at: http://ipal.capc.org/downloads/ipal-icu-defining-standards-for-icu-palliative-care.pdf. Published July 2010. Accessed September 22, 2013.
3. Aslakson RA, Bridges JF. Assess the impact of palliative care in the intensive care unit through the leans of patient-centered outcomes research. Curr Opin Crit Care 2013;19:504–10. http://dx.doi.org/10.1097/MCC.0b013e328364d50f.
4. Ferrell BR, Dablin C, Campbell ML, et al. End-of-Life Nursing Education Consortium (ELNEC) Training Program: improving palliative care in critical care. Crit

Care Nurs Q 2007;30:206–12. http://dx.doi.org/10.1097/01.CNQ.0000278920. 37068.e9.

5. Levin TT, Moreno B, Silvester W, et al. End of life communication in the intensive care unit. Gen Hosp Psychiatry 2010;32:433–42. http://dx.doi.org/10.1016/j. genhosppsych.2010.04.007.

6. Grossman S. Development of the palliative care of dying critically ill patients algorithm. J Hosp Palliat Nurs 2013;15:355–9.

7. Camhi SL, Mercado AF, Morrison SR, et al. Deciding in the dark: advanced directives and continuation of treatment in chronic critical illness. Crit Care Med 2009; 37:919–25. http://dx.doi.org/10.1097/CCM.06013e31819613cc.

8. Loertscher L, Reed DA, Bannon MP, et al. Cardiopulmonary resuscitation and do not resuscitate orders: a guide for clinicians. Am J Med 2010;123:4–9. http://dx. doi.org/10.1016/j.amjmed.2009.05.029.

9. Kass-Bartelems BL, Hughes R. Advanced care planning, preferences for care at the end of life: research in action. Agency for Healthcare Research and Quality. Available at: http://www.ahrq.gov/research/findings/factsheets/aging/endliferia/ index.html. Published March 2003. Accessed September 9, 2013.

10. Penrod JD, Deb P, Dellenbaugh C, et al. Hospital based palliative care consultation: effects on hospital cost. J Palliat Med 2010;13:973–9. http://dx.doi.org/10. 1089/jpm.2010.0038.

11. Connors AF, Dawson NV, Desbien NA, et al. A controlled trial to improve care for seriously ill hospitalized patients. JAMA 1995;274:1591–8.

12. Resnick B. Ethics and medical futility: the healthcare professional's role. Presented at the National Conference of Gerontological Nurse Practitioners (NCGNP) 25th Annual Meeting. Ponte Vedra Beach (FL), September 27–October 1, 2006.

13. Raphael C, Ahrens J, Fowler N. Financing end of life care in the USA. J R Soc Med 2001;94:458–61. Available at: http://www.ncbi.nlm.nih.gov/pmc/articles/ PMC1282187/pdf/0940458.pdf.

14. Lubitz JD, Riley GF. Trends in Medicare payments in the last year of life. N Engl J Med 1993;328:1092–6. http://dx.doi.org/10.1056/NEJM199304153281506.

15. Mosenthal AC, Weissman DE, Curtis JR, et al. Integrating palliative care in the surgical and trauma intensive care unit: a report from the Improving Palliative Care in the Intensive Care Unit (IPAL-ICU) Project Advisory Board and the Center to Advance Palliative Care. Crit Care Med 2012;40:1199–206. http://dx.doi.org/ 10.1097/CCm.0b013e31823bc8e7.

16. Nelson JE, Puntillo KA, Pronovost PJ, et al. In their own words: patients and families define high-quality palliative care in the intensive care unit. Crit Care Med 2010;38:808–18. http://dx.doi.org/10.1097/CCm.0b013e3181c5887c.

17. Strand JJ, Billings JA. Integrating palliative care in the intensive care unit. J Support Oncol 2012;10(5):180–7.

18. Begun JW, Zimmerman B, Dooley K. Healthcare organizations as complex adaptive systems. In: Mick SE, Wyttenchach M, editors. Advances in health care organization theory. San Francisco (CA): Jossey-Bass; 2008. p. 253–88.

Driving Hospital-Acquired Pressure Ulcers to Zero

Donna Morehead, MSN/INF, RN, NE-BC*, Brenda Blain, DNP, RN, FACHE, NEA-BC

KEYWORDS

- Hospital-acquired pressure ulcers • Unit-acquired pressure ulcers
- Intensive care unit • Staff nurse accountability • Change process
- NDNQI pressure ulcer education • Bedside report • Braden score

KEY POINTS

- Pressure ulcer formation in the ICU is no longer acceptable.
- Yearly competencies for identification of pressure ulcers may be the key to eliminating hospital-acquired pressure ulcers.
- Stage I pressure ulcers must be identified accurately to stop the progression to open wounds.
- When bedside RNs are given the task of solving problems, positive outcomes occur.
- Collaborative bedside report creates accountability.

A patient admitted into the intensive care unit (ICU) may have a single or even multiple organs failing; be sustained on life-saving equipment, such as ventilators; and is usually hemodynamically unstable and maintained on vasoactive drugs, which divert oxygen-rich blood flow from extremities to major organs. All of these issues make the ICU patient a prime candidate for the development of a pressure ulcer.[1] Because of these issues, many ICU nurses believed that pressure ulcers in the ICU could not be avoided. The issue is to change the mindset, hold individuals accountable, and have a goal of zero pressure ulcers. The new thought needs to be that pressure ulcers are preventable.

Pressure ulcers have mental, physical, and financial implications for the individual and the organization. A loss of confidence in the organization can occur when a patient develops any hospital-acquired condition. Patient and family expectations are focused on healing or maintaining health care issues, not the development of new health care concerns during their hospitalization. Physically, the development of hospital-acquired pressure ulcers creates discomfort and body image distortion while requiring additional treatments and medications. In the world of health care, the

The authors have nothing to disclose.
Baylor Medical Center at Irving, 1901 N. MacArthur, Irving, TX 75061, USA
* Corresponding author.
E-mail address: DonnaMor@baylorhealth.edu

financial implications related to hospital-acquired pressure ulcers have a major impact on a hospital's financial outcome. Each pressure ulcer can add a cost ranging from $2384 to $17,495 per case.[2]

The prevention of hospital-acquired pressure ulcers remains a top priority for health care facilities worldwide. This article discusses a process improvement in an ICU where the unit-acquired pressure ulcer rate was dropped from 30% to 0% by front-line staff nurses. The key areas addressed by the staff were education, creating a process for turning patients during bedside report, and the creation of a documentation tool for accurate skin/wound assessment. Involving front-line staff in the prevention methodology creates a process that is quickly adopted by staff, peer-to-peer accountability in accurate skin/wound assessment, and positive outcomes.

LITERATURE REVIEW

To prevent an event from happening, one must understand why it occurs. The literature is rich with research on pressure ulcers, their potential causes, and possible solutions. However, one research study tends to contradict another. For example, a patient's gender has been identified as a potential risk factor in obtaining a pressure ulcer. A study conducted by Compton and colleagues[3] identified males as having a significantly higher rate of pressure ulcers, whereas other studies found females were at higher risk[4,5]; however, another study did not find gender to be a factor.[6] Age was also identified as a potential predictor of obtaining a pressure ulcer. In several studies patients older than 65 years of age were identified as being at a higher risk of developing a pressure ulcer,[4,7,8] yet a study completed in Tokyo found, when looking at pressure ulcer development, age was not a risk factor.[9]

Another contradictory factor discussed in the literature is body weight and body mass. Although obese patients have been identified as having a higher risk of pressure ulcers while hospitalized,[3,10,11] body mass was not a valuable variable because of fluid accumulation and body wasting that occurs in the ICU.[6,11]

In some studies, nutritional status within the ICU is also a potential contributor of pressure ulcers. Because of the level of illness, feeding patients is frequently delayed, which can create a loss of subcutaneous tissue and can increase pressure on bony prominences, thereby increasing the risk of a pressure ulcer.[12] However, the laboratory data usually used in identifying a patient's nutritional status, such as serum albumin and protein, do not show statistically significant differences in patients that developed pressure ulcers compared with those patients that did not.[6]

More consistent risk factors in the literature associated with pressure ulcers include patients with multiple chronic illnesses, especially vascular disease and congestive heart failure; patients with low arterial and systolic pressure; and patients receiving vasopressors.[4,7,10,11,13-15] The consistent reasoning for this was a lack of oxygen and nutrients to the capillary beds that supply the skin.

As previously noted, the literature is full of contradictory information about pressure ulcers and their potential physiologic causes. Within the intensive care setting, additional issues also exist that can contribute to the increased risk of pressure ulcers. If a patient is intubated, or has a tube feeding infusing, the head of the bed is elevated to prevent aspiration. This elevation increases the risk of shearing and friction, which contributes to pressure ulcer development.[6,7,12] Nurses within the intensive care should also consider the length of time the patient may have been laying on a surgical, ambulance, or hospital stretcher awaiting testing and admission.[4,9]

All of these issues could help explain why a patient in the ICU is twice as likely to leave the unit with a pressure ulcer as is a patient in the acute care setting.[14,15]

Because pressure ulcers increase discomfort for the patient, cost for the hospital, and length of stay,[2,5,10,11,13,14] it is important that the ICU staff identify innovative ways to incorporate prevention of pressure ulcers in their daily practice. Currently, there does not seem to be one tool that can adequately predict individuals that will develop a pressure ulcer in the ICU.[14,16] To prevent pressure ulcers in the ICU, a team approach needs to occur, evaluating the patient frequently, and changing the plan of care as the patient's condition changes, which can be frequent in this type of setting.[4,6,7,9,16]

CHANGE PROCESS

In 2007, the ICU at Baylor Medical Center at Irving had a pressure ulcer issue. The unit had a 30% unit-acquired pressure ulcer rate, as reported by the National Database for Nursing Quality Indicators (NDNQI). To fix the issue, it was obvious staff had to be a part of the solution. In a unit staff meeting the pressure ulcer data were discussed and the staff were asked if the numbers were acceptable to them. The nursing staff stated that pressure ulcers were something that occurred in the ICU, but agreed the number could be improved. The staff nurses decided to form a team and tackle the problem.

The team was asked to research current evidence-based practices and to bring their articles and ideas to the first team meeting. In the first meeting, the discussion was focused on what they had learned in their literature search. The team identified turning practices; pressure ulcer risk scoring, such as the Braden Scale; specialty beds with pressure-reducing surfaces; and the use of skin/wound specialists. The interesting part was that the team believed that each of these items were already in place within our facility, yet we had a recognized issue that needed solutions.

Using their new found information, the team identified the potential reasons for the high rates of unit-acquired pressure ulcers. The areas the team believed needed work were (1) lack of knowledge concerning pressure ulcer identification, (2) time required for turning patients, and (3) documentation of skin/wound issues.

EDUCATION

Because education was identified as the highest priority need, the team decided an education program to assist the staff in accurately identifying pressure ulcers would be created. The team all agreed that it was easy to see and identify stage II and greater pressure ulcers, but staff would tend to miss the stage I pressure ulcers or attribute them to laying on a stretcher for prolonged periods of time and believed they would resolve themselves. The team researched different education programs and decided to use the NDNQI program for pressure ulcer identification. All staff nurses in the ICU were required to complete the education program. The wound and skin experts from the physical therapy department were asked to join the ICU team as adjunct team members. These experts assisted the nursing staff in identifying educational opportunities, supported the nursing staff as they took on this process, and remained invested stakeholders in this process by offering their consulting services to any staff member with questions concerning staging pressure ulcers. Over the next 3 years new employees were required to complete the NDNQI education program so that all ICU staff were competent in pressure ulcer identification. Staff were held accountable for the NDNQI education program by printing and turning in the certificate of completion.

The education program provided great results. The unit had zero pressure ulcers until the second quarter of 2011. A stage II pressure ulcer was found in the ICU. This devastated the staff and triggered the team to reevaluate the staffs' knowledge on pressure ulcers. When the team learned that education was lacking again, they decided it was important to require the staff to complete the NDNQI education on a yearly basis as a competency.

TURNING PATIENTS

The team also looked at issues surrounding barriers in turning patients. The team believed that tasks stole their time and made it difficult to turn patients, especially at the beginning and end of their shifts. As they looked at the work flow, it was noted that as the end of the shift got closer, the nurse would complete their turning tasks about 1 hour before the end of the shift to improve the efficiency of the hand-off report time. The oncoming shift, especially the day shift, found that the beginning of their shift was filled with physicians rounding, and such tasks as discontinuation of chest tubes, pulling of critical lines, or other physician-initiated tasks, that would keep them busy and delay them from turning patients in a timely manner. This resulted in some patients going as long as 4 hours without being turned. To meet patient needs, the staff nurses decided to create a practice change and turn the patients and complete a skin assessment during their bedside hand-off report. This process change solved two issues: it provided the nursing staff with a second pair of eyes while assessing the skin as they became more comfortable with their assessment skills; and it gave the nursing staff the number of people needed to turn patients efficiently and in a timely manner. With all patients in the ICU being turned between 7:00 and 7:30 AM or PM, the entire interdisciplinary team was knowledgeable of patient turning times. This also established the turning schedule for all staff during their shift. Over time, the nursing staff expanded the bedside shift report to include a quick shift assessment; identification of lines, tubes, and drains; and other infection-prevention methodology assessments. This was a huge step for the staff on the unit. The staff became accountable to each other, which not only helped with pressure ulcers but also improved the change of shift process. No longer were staff allowed to leave an empty or almost empty bag of intravenous fluids, dirty linen, unkempt rooms, or nonfunctioning intravenous lines.

DOCUMENTATION

Documentation issues were also identified with our computer-based documentation system. This system was implemented in the 1990s and was a very good system, but the software was outdated. The system lacked the ability to retrieve documentation without printing out all nursing documentation from admission to current date. For several years the night shift unit technicians would print out the prior days documentation for the nurse to review the patient's skin history. Because of cost saving initiatives, this process was deleted and the practice stopped. The nursing staff had no way to see the prior shift's documentation. The system also made it difficult to compare the current assessment with previous assessments. The vital sign graphic sheets had remained on paper with this computer system so the staff recreated the graphic sheet as a trifold document and added the new skin/wound assessment to the paper form (**Fig. 1**). This paper tool required the staff to document the presence of skin/wound issues. To push the accountability to the bedside the on-coming and off-going registered nurses (RNs) were responsible for signing the tool to verify that they agreed with the assessment and that the assessment took place. In August of 2012 the organization implemented a new electronic health record. The new documentation no longer had the image of the human anatomy but the staff found no difficulty in using the new system for documentation. The documentation is easily followed with each shift's assessment lining up side by side for comparison. The process of bedside

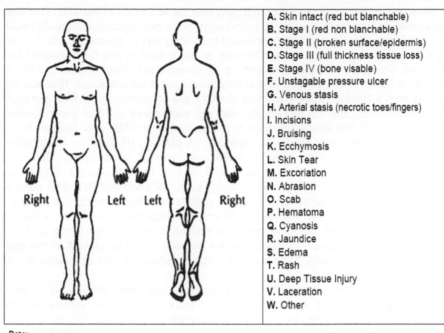

A. Skin intact (red but blanchable)
B. Stage I (red non blanchable)
C. Stage II (broken surface/epidermis)
D. Stage III (full thickness tissue loss)
E. Stage IV (bone visable)
F. Unstagable pressure ulcer
G. Venous stasis
H. Arterial stasis (necrotic toes/fingers)
I. Incisions
J. Bruising
K. Ecchymosis
L. Skin Tear
M. Excoriation
N. Abrasion
O. Scab
P. Hematoma
Q. Cyanosis
R. Jaundice
S. Edema
T. Rash
U. Deep Tissue Injury
V. Laceration
W. Other

Right   Left   Left   Right

Date: _____

| Special Therapy Mattress_____ | Skin Consult _____ | Nutritional Consult _____ |

Time	Wound #	Type	Size	Comments

Shift Initials Signature   Shift Initials Signature

BAYLOR MEDICAL CENTER AT IRVING

SKIN / WOUND ASSESSMENT FORM
X-XXX   PAGE 1 OF 1   PS2554 (02/25/08)

PLACE PATIENT LABEL HERE

Fig. 1. Skin/wound assessment form.

assessment had been hardwired with the nursing staff for several years and continued seamlessly without the written verification of the bedside report.

Administrative support was essential in this project with the chief nursing officer attending many of the unit meetings. When the staff discussed the literature they found on surfaces and beds in the ICU, the chief nursing officer contacted the facility supplier for beds and found three reconditioned specialty beds for use in the ICU. This idea was enthusiastically accepted by the team but posed a new problem for the ICU staff. How would they decide which patient would be placed on the specialty beds. Ninety-five percent of the patients in the ICU were at some level of risk for pressure ulcer formation. The team decided to complete a retrospective chart review to identify the Braden Scale scores of patients that had developed pressure ulcers. Traditionally, patients with a Braden Scale score less than 18 are considered at risk for pressure ulcer development. But not all patients with a Braden score of 18 or lower develop pressure ulcers.[17] The Braden Scale was first published in 1987 and consists of six sections: (1) sensory perception, (2) moisture, (3) activity, (4) mobility, (5) nutrition, and (6) friction and shearing. Five risk levels are identified in the Braden Scale: (1) very high for a score of less than or equal to 9, (2) high risk has a score of 10 to 12, (3) moderate risk is 13 to 14, (4) low risk is 15 to 18, and (5) a score of 19 to 23 is considered no risk. The team went back through all patients that had developed a pressure ulcer in the ICU for the previous year and found that they consistently had a Braden score of 15 or less. The team decided that patients with a Braden score of 15 or less and if they were unable to tolerate active mobility would be placed on the specialty bed or if no specialty beds were available, a specialty bed or overlay would be rented.

Throughout this process, monthly meetings were conducted with the team members to discuss the project and outcomes. Each team member was held responsible to discuss ongoing changes that needed to be implemented in the ICU for ongoing reduction of unit-acquired pressure ulcers and the rational for those changes.

BARRIERS IDENTIFIED

The two barriers identified during this process improvement project included noncompliance with the education and resistance to change. Noncompliance was addressed by giving deadlines for completion of the education programs and holding staff accountable. The staff were given 2 weeks to complete the education program. If the staff chose to not complete the education program a verbal discussion took place with the manager at the 2-week mark. If continued noncompliance was an issue then the disciplinary process was followed with written opportunities for improvement and expectations that were clear for the staff member to understand the expectations. Thankfully only two staff members required this extra guidance. To address resistance, the manager and charge RN visually monitored bedside report the first week of implementation. In the second week on-coming and off-going staff RNs were held accountable for signing the wound and skin assessment by ICU team members auditing the documentation daily. Peer-to-peer accountability started with verbal reminders. In a few cases, some staff needed formal work improvement plans to promote the change process. Change is difficult for everyone and this process change was no exception. Some of the staff were concerned that the new process would increase the time that report would take. The team worked hard to reassure the staff that even though shift report may take a bit longer, the increase in accurate information concerning the patient would be worth the time and allow for better patient outcomes. The number of staff that remained resistant to the changes in report was minimal and peer-to-peer accountability became the key. Eventually, staff refused to sign the skin/wound assessment documentation if bedside assessment did not take place. Cosignatures were a required element with the team auditing to ensure that each shift followed the new process. When a cosignature was not found, the staff were questioned as to why this process had not taken place. Verbal reminders were used along with re-education of why this new process was important. Each day the verbal reminders were fewer and within 2 weeks, this process was adopted by all staff.

In the second quarter of 2011 the ICU had its first pressure ulcer in more than 3 years (**Fig. 2**). The same team reunited to identify new potential issues. Every area of patient care was evaluated to see what had been missed. The one item that had not been evaluated thoroughly was the unit mattresses. The staff researched to determine the age of the mattresses and the life expectancy of the mattresses. The mattresses were noted to be close to 10 years old with a life expectancy of 7 to 8 years. New mattresses were purchased for all beds within the ICU. With the change of the mattresses, the unit-acquired pressure ulcer rate dropped back to zero.

PRACTICAL APPLICATION

One of the most challenging issues with pressure ulcer assessment is accurate identification of stage I pressure ulcers. Unstageable and stage II or greater pressure ulcers are easily noted with identifiable open wounds, whereas stage I pressure ulcers may have little color change or appear red and are quickly attributed to the patient lying on an area for a prolonged period of time. Deep tissue injuries are easy to indentify but are frequently dismissed as a simple burse that will heal without difficulty. Unless properly assessed, these areas are overlooked and the perfect opportunity for prevention methods missed. Vigilance in accurately identifying and documenting pressure ulcers must be a priority. The ICU posts nursing quality indicator reports including unit-acquired pressure ulcers on a bulletin board at the entrance of the ICU for all staff, patients, and visitors to see. Current rates are discussed weekly in the 7:00 AM unit huddle, which includes day and night shift nursing staff.

Appropriate education in assessing stage I pressure ulcers is the key to preventing advancement of pressure ulcers. With proper prevention techniques, such as frequent turning and specialized air mattresses, stage I pressure ulcers can be reversed with little cost to the health care facility. Each time a patient is turned, or returns from such areas as dialysis, radiology, or surgery, these areas must be meticulously examined for stage I pressure ulcers by trained staff. Radiology and surgery are two areas where patients are required to lay on hard surfaces for prolonged periods, creating the perfect scenarios for pressure ulcer formation. Yearly competencies for the proper identification of pressure ulcers is necessary and creates a solid knowledge base for nursing staff to identify and prevent pressure ulcers. Nursing accountability and ownership of the issues within their environment is an important piece to this puzzle. Top-down process changes are frequently short lived because problems associated

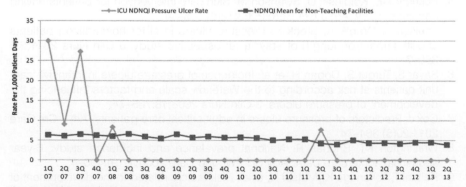

Fig. 2. Baylor Medical Center at Irving ICU unit-acquired pressure ulcer rate.

with the process are poorly understood. Creating a bottom-up process change by engaging, encouraging, and supporting the bedside nursing staff in finding solutions that work within their environment creates a successful process change. Accurate documentation of pressure ulcers and skin issues remains a challenge. Determining if a pressure ulcer is present on admission or was hospital-acquired can be a daunting task, and when missed, a financial burden to the health care facility. Two key elements assist with documentation: a documentation system that enhances accurate assessment elements; and house-wide education to create uniformity of documentation. Scheduled audits are useful to ensure accurate documentation, especially when the front-line staff is engaged in this process.

SUMMARY

The application of the understanding of health care as a complex adaptive system involves cultivating an environment of listening to people, enhancing relationships, and allowing creative ideas to emerge by creating small nonthreatening changes that attract and retain excellent individuals.[18] Change is never permanent, it requires constant vigilance. Driving the unit-acquired pressure ulcer rate to zero certainly fits this category. The ICU staff recognized unit-acquired pressure ulcers as a problematic area and identified three areas for change: (1) education, (2) turning patients, and (3) documentation. The key to the success of this change process is involving staff nurses from the start, staff empowerment, and peer-to-peer accountability throughout the process. Achieving zero was not as difficult as maintaining the pressure ulcer occurrence rate at zero. It is unrealistic to believe that this unit will maintain a zero unit-acquired pressure ulcer rate permanently. What is realistic is to keep the focus on the data and strive to achieve the best possible outcome for each individual patient in our care.

REFERENCES

1. Curry K, Kutash M, Chambers H. A prospective, descriptive study of characteristics associated with ski failure in critically ill adults. Ostomy Wound Manage 2012;68(5):36–43.
2. Beckrich K, Aronovitch SA. Hospital-acquired pressure ulcers: a comparison of costs in medical vs. surgical patients. Nurs Econ 1999;17(5):263–71.
3. Compton F, Hoffmann F, Hortig T, et al. Pressure ulcer predictors in ICU patients: nursing skin assessment versus objective parameters. J Wound Care 2008; 17(10):417–20.
4. Pokorny ME, Koldjeski D, Swanson M. Skin care intervention for patients having cardiac surgery. Am J Crit Care 2003;12(6):535–44.
5. Theisen S, Drabik A, Stock S. Pressure ulcers in older hospitalized patients and its impact on length of stay: a retrospective study. J Clin Nurs 2011;21: 380–7.
6. Sayar S, Turgut S, Dogan H, et al. Incidence of pressure ulcers in intensive care unit patients at risk according to the Waterlow scale and factors influencing the development of pressure ulcers. J Clin Nurs 2008;18:765–74.
7. Cox J. Predictors of pressure ulcers in adult critical care patients. Am J Crit Care 2011;20(5):364–74.
8. Whittington KT, Briones R. National prevalence and incidence study: 6-year sequential acute care data. Adv Skin Wound Care 2004;17(9):490–4.
9. Kaitani T, Tokunaga K, Matsui N, et al. Risk factors related to the development of pressure ulcers in the critical care setting. J Clin Nurs 2010;19:414–21.

10. Lyder CH, Wang Y, Metersky M, et al. Hospital-acquired pressure ulcers: results from the national Medicare patient safety monitoring system study. J Am Geriatr Soc 2012;60:1603–8.
11. Theaker C, Mannan M, Ives N, et al. Risk factors for pressure sores in the critically ill. Anaesthesia 2000;55:221–4.
12. Estilo ME, Angeles A, Perez T, et al. Pressure ulcers in the intensive care unit: new perspectives on an old problem. Crit Care Nurse 2012;32(3):65–70.
13. Graves N, Birrell F, Whitby M. Effect of pressure ulcers on length of hospital stay. Infect Control Hosp Epidemiol 2005;26(3):293–7.
14. Keller PJ, Ville J, van Ramshorst B, et al. Pressure ulcers in intensive care patients: a review of risks and prevention. Intensive Care Med 2002;28:1379–88.
15. Nijs N, Toppets A, Defloor T, et al. Incidence and risk factors for pressure ulcers in the intensive care unit. J Clin Nurs 2008;18:1258–66.
16. Stotts NA, Wu HS. Hospital recovery is facilitated by prevention of pressure ulcers in older adults. Crit Care Nurs Clin North Am 2007;19:269–75.
17. Bergstrom N, Braden BJ, Laquzza A. The Braden Scale for predicting pressure sore risk. Nurse Res 1987;36(4):205–10.
18. Holden LM. Complex adaptive systems: concept analysis. J Adv Nurs 2005; 52(6):651–7.

Fall Prevention in High-Risk Patients

Kathleen M. Shuey, MS, RN, AOCN, ACNS-BC[a],*, Christine Balch, RN, BSN, OCN[b]

KEYWORDS

- Fall • Accidental fall • Prevention • Oncology • High Risk

KEY POINTS

- Implement a bundle approach using a multidisciplinary team to promote patient safety.
- Consistent, purposeful hourly rounding is one program element that can provide an immediate impact on reduction of falls.
- Disease process and treatment factors place oncology patients at an increased risk of fall and subsequent injury.

INTRODUCTION

In 2012, the Centers for Disease Control and Prevention reported that 28.3% of nonfatal injuries in all age groups were due to falls.[1] The National Database for Nursing Quality Indicators (NDNQI) defines a fall as an unplanned decent to any surface.[2] In the United States, unintentional falls, in the community and health care setting, are the leading cause of nonfatal injury. Approximately 26,000 deaths are attributed to unintentional falls resulting in a cost of approximately $30 billion.[3] In the past, the additional medical care cost for a fall was passed on to the patient and payor. The Center for Medicare and Medicaid Services (CMS) no longer reimburses hospitals for additional expenses resulting from a fall. Insurers may follow the lead of CMS on reimbursement.

In the health care setting, nursing is responsible for identifying at-risk patients and populations; educating the patient, family members, and clinical staff of associated risks; and implementing prevention measures. Several fall-prevention tools are available that facilitate nursing assessment and identify patients at risk for falls. Based on the risk score of the individual tool, nursing can implement patient-specific

Funding Sources: Nil.

Conflict of Interest: Nil.

[a] Department of Nursing, Oncology, Baylor University Medical Center at Dallas, T. Boone Pickens Cancer Hospital, 5th Floor, 3535 Worth Street, Dallas, TX 75246, USA; [b] Department of Nursing, Baylor University Medical Center at Dallas, T. Boone Pickens Cancer Hospital, 5th Floor, 3535 Worth Street, Dallas, TX 75246, USA

* Corresponding author.

E-mail address: kathleen.shuey@baylorhealth.edu

interventions to prevent fall events. However, fall-prevention tools are just one component of a comprehensive fall-prevention safety program. Falls remain one of the top adverse events in hospitalized patients.

REVIEW OF LITERATURE

In the prevention of falls, there is no one key intervention that will impact overall incidence. The literature supports a bundle approach using a multidisciplinary team to promote patient safety.[4–6] The Agency for Healthcare Research and Quality has developed a toolkit, Preventing Falls in Hospitals, which provides a step-by-step guide for implementation of an evidence-based fall-prevention program.[7] Elements of a comprehensive fall-prevention program include support of senior leadership at the facility, assessment of current practices, identification of team members, implementation of interventions, and follow-up of events (**Box 1**).

Patient characteristics that influence risk for falls include change in mental status/cognition, muscle strength, mobility, and fatigue.[8,9] Age, gender, medical diagnosis, and severity of illness are variables that have not been found to have an impact on prevention of falls.[8]

After selecting a fall-risk tool, interventions should be tailored to the various risk levels within the tool. Because of the bundled approach to fall prevention, the impact of a single intervention on fall prevention cannot be assessed. However, several authors mention the positive impact of hourly rounding.[6,10–12] One study noted a decrease in call-light utilization when hourly rounding was implemented.[11] Purposeful rounding promotes a proactive approach to assessment of the patient and environment of care.

Polypharmacy is often cited as a factor in falls. One analysis suggests that the category of medication (benzodiazepines, barbiturates, antidepressants, antiemetics, and psychotropic agents) leads to the increase in risk versus the number of medications.[6,8,13] Patients may experience dizziness, drowsiness, confusion, or loss of balance as a result of select medications. Increased urgency for toileting is implicated

---

Box 1
Key elements of a fall-prevention program

- Support of hospital leadership and identification of key stakeholders.
- Assessment of current state and identification of needed resources.
- Identification of an interdisciplinary team.
- Determination of the best practices.
- Implementation of hospital/unit best practice/interventions (eg, scheduled rounding, assessment of environmental safety).
- Implementation of patient-specific best practice/interventions (eg, use of a fall-prevention risk assessment tool, medication evaluation tool, delirium assessment, mobilization protocol, and patient-specific education).
- Implement an after-fall review and root cause analysis.
- Assessment, development, and implementation an orientation/education program for hospital staff (clinical and nonclinical).

Data from Agency for Healthcare Research and Quality. Preventing falls in hospitals: a toolkit for improving quality of care. Available at: http://www.ahrq.gov/professionals/systems/hospital/fallpxtoolkit/fallpxtoolkit.pdf. Accessed February 22, 2014.

in the use of antidiarrheal and laxative-type agents.[6] Anticoagulants do not increase fall risk but may have an impact on the extent of the injury due to coagulation issues. Working collaboratively with the pharmacist can facilitate early identification of problematic side effects and potential medication interactions.

Locating the patient at risk closer to the nursing station and use of sitters allow direct visualization of the patient and patient room.[6,14–16] Conflicting information on use of bed and chair alarms, low rise beds, and bevel-edged mats during the night while patients are sleeping on overall fall reduction is noted in the literature.[6,19] However, these devices can decrease the severity of injury if a fall occurs.

Patients who are hospitalized may become debilitated over time because of the actual illness or as a result of prolonged inactivity. Preventative interventions, such as range of motion or isometric exercises, ambulating, and Physical Therapy consultations, can enhance mobility, strength, and endurance.[4,9] Webcams are another tool that may assist in decreasing falls. Hardin and colleagues noted that patients initially were apprehensive about the lack of privacy while nursing staff expressed concern over monitoring of nursing activity via the Webcam.[18] The study determined that, although not statistically significant, fewer falls occurred at the intervention hospital when the Webcam was used.

One hospital described the impact of patient feedback on interventions that were implemented by the hospital fall team.[17] Effectiveness of interventions were graded as weak, medium, and strong. The patient participant identified environmental factors that had a strong impact on the hospital fall program. Education and policy changes were categorized as weak, having little impact, while checklists and enhanced communication between staff had a moderate impact on fall rates.

Development of a comprehensive education plan should focus on both clinical and nonclinical staff.[12,18] Orientation to the hospital and inpatient unit should include discussion of facility safety programs including fall prevention.[12,18] Instruction on the use of patient-specific equipment, such as gait belts, bed alarms, and lift equipment, will increase the technical competency of staff promoting a culture of safety.

Although there is little mention of the impact of staffing or level of staff on falls, Titler and colleagues[8] noted that an increase in the RN skill mix by 10% was significantly associated with decreased falls during hospitalization. Critical thinking is a key element in the decision-making process and is essential to the prevention of falls.

Oncology Patient Characteristics

A review of oncology-specific literature revealed 2 areas of focus: description of patient characteristics and interventional studies. Patient-related risk factors are similar to the general population and include fatigue, immobility, inappropriate footwear, poor illumination, and inattention to surroundings. Predictors of ongoing fall risk include presence of cancer-related pain syndrome, daily dose of benzodiazepine, and severity of depression.[19] Of interest, oncology patients who had a serious injury were found in one study to have fewer medical comorbidities than the general population.[20] Additional characteristics that may be associated with falls include functional status, treatment (chemotherapy, biotherapy, surgery, radiation therapy, or endocrine therapy), depression, blood administration, anemia, and nutritional status.[13]

Treatment-related patient factors include balance disturbances, such as peripheral neuropathy, a side effect of select chemotherapy agents.[21] Visual disturbances have been documented in women undergoing treatment with endocrine therapy.[21,22] Men receiving androgen deprivation therapy (ADT) experienced more falls when compared with a similar group.[23] The exact mechanism of action is unknown. However, androgen deprivation induces a mild anemia that can lead to increased fatigue.

Long-term treatment with ADT can decrease bone mineral density, potentially contributing to fall risk. Corticosteroid-induced myopathy, antiemetic therapy, and pain management also contribute to an increased risk of falls.[19,20]

Disease-related factors include metastatic disease and hematologic diagnosis requiring bone marrow transplantation.[19,20] Patients with primary brain tumors or metastases are twice as likely to fall as patients without cerebral involvement.[19]

Overcash and Beckstead[24] prospectively evaluated oncology patients 70 years and older using a Comprehensive Geriatric Assessment that included Activities of Daily Living Scale, Instructional Activities of Daily Living Scale (IADL), Geriatric Depression Scale, and Mini-Mental State Examination. The IADL scale, which addresses factors such as the ability to use the telephone, shop, prepare food, handle finances, and be responsible for medications, was found to predict falls. An inverse relationship was noted, as the score decreased, the risk of fall increased.

Lower level of pain, presence of metastatic disease, use of antidepressants and antipsychotics, and weak or impaired gait predicted an increased fall risk of hospitalized patients.[25] One study indicated that duration of hospitalization is positively correlated with falls.[26] As length of stay increased, fall risk also increased.

Interventions in the Oncology Population

Progressive weight-training, weight-bearing exercises, and interventions targeted toward improved balance and range of motion were found to improve lower extremity strength and balance.[27] Strength training has a positive impact on patients with diabetic peripheral neuropathy and holds promise for those patients experiencing chemotherapy-induced neuropathy.[27]

A nurse-directed exercise program, Moving to Wellness, demonstrated an 81% improvement or maintenance of muscle strength score.[28] The program was developed collaboratively by a multidisciplinary group that included nurses, physicians, and physical therapists. The exercise plan was based on the patient's functional status providing 3 exercise options.

Patient-focused and family-focused education can enhance knowledge of fall risk, promote safe mobility, and conceivably prevent falls. A DVD program, Moving Safely in the Home, was found to increase individual perception about safe mobility and fall prevention.[29] After viewing the DVD, a significant increase of fall-prevention knowledge was found in a convenience sample of family caregivers for individuals with a variety of cancers. The DVD was viewed on average at least twice during the study. The overall fall-risk score was significantly lower at 3 months after viewing the DVD than before the study. Six falls were reported in the 3 months preceding the study. No falls were reported in the 4-month follow-up period.

QUALITY IMPROVEMENT PROJECT

A 32-bed and 24-bed inpatient medical oncology unit at a 500+ bed hospital located in a large metropolitan area of the south was experiencing elevated fall and fall with injury rates. A quality improvement project was initiated on the units to decrease falls and falls with injury. Data from 7 of the 11 quarters before project implementation indicated that falls were greater than the 50th percentile when compared with comparable units in the NDNQI. A team of clinical staff (including RNs and patient care technicians) initially met to identify steps in determining fall risk (**Fig. 1**). The project facilitator then met with nursing staff across all shifts to identify issues that contributed to falls. Identified issues were grouped into 4 categories: people (bed alarm becomes white noise, inconsistent rounding), patient/family (age, independence, confusion, deconditioning),

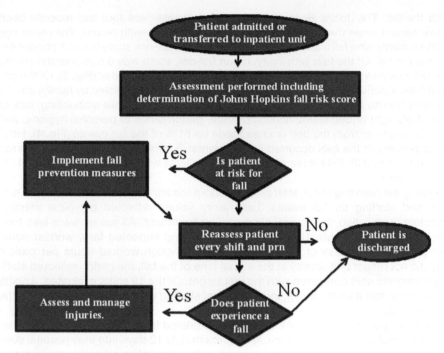

Fig. 1. Steps in determining fall risk.

environment (equipment, signage), and lack of understanding by patient family of risk (**Fig. 2**).

Falls occurring in a 4-month time frame from May 2011 through August 2011 were reviewed to evaluate trends and identify patient characteristics. A total of 19 falls occurred, approximately one fall every 6.5 days. Of the falls, 4 patients had an injury

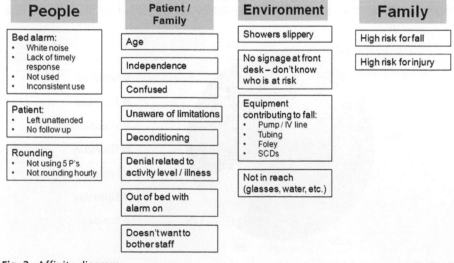

Fig. 2. Affinity diagram.

with the fall. The Johns Hopkins Hospital Fall Assessment tool had recently been implemented when the units began using an electronic health record. The mean age of the patients who fell was 63. Mean Johns Hopkins fall-risk score was 7.8 (moderate) before the fall. Of the falls with injury, mean fall-risk score was 6.5 (moderate) before the fall. Forty-two percent of falls occurred on a Tuesday or Friday (**Fig. 3**). Of the patient falls, 4 patients were assisted by staff, 4 patients were assisted by family, and 11 patients had no assistance during the event. Falls occurring while ambulating, lack of use of call light or bed alarm, noncompliance, performance of personal hygiene, and transferring to or from the bed or chair made up 81% of the fall events (**Fig. 4**). Fifty-three percent of the falls occurred on the nightshift, while 47% of the falls occurred during the dayshift. Fifty-three percent of the patients who fell were men, while 47% were women.

During the planning cycle, staff inquired about the impact of treatment-related factors and staffing on fall events. Laboratory values reflected a typical medical oncology population that is actively receiving treatment. All values were less than the normal range (**Table 1**). To determine if staffing impacted falls, worked hours per patient day on day of fall were analyzed. Although worked hours per patient day did not reflect unit activity at the actual time of the fall, the metric reflected staffing during the shift compared with the unit target. Of the 19 shifts evaluated, 4 shifts (21%) were less than the target, indicating that staffing was not a factor in 79% of the falls (**Fig. 5**).

One unexpected outcome of the project was related to length of stay. Data analysis identified that patients, on average, fell approximately 12 days into their hospital stay. Medical oncology patients enter the hospital with a good physical performance status before starting therapy. During the course of hospitalization, patients become debilitated possibly due to disease process, treatment factors (such as low hemoglobin/hematocrit and red blood cell count), or immobility (a result of prolonged hospitalization). The patient may not readily recognize that his or her performance status has deteriorated and continue to act independently.

CASE STUDY

The patient, a 58-year-old man, was admitted with a new diagnosis of acute myelogenous leukemia. The patient arrived ambulatory accompanied by his wife. He was

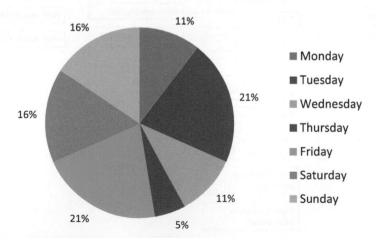

Fig. 3. Percentage of falls by day of week.

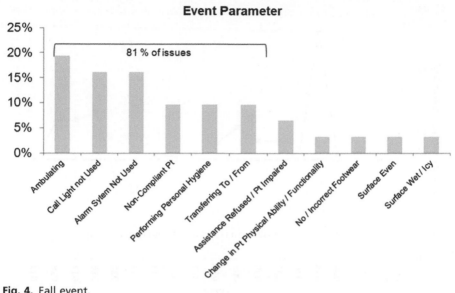

Fig. 4. Fall event.

transferred from a facility approximately 200 miles away for treatment. His wife planned to stay with him around the clock on the inpatient unit.

On the second day of his hospital stay, the patient received induction chemotherapy. During his nadir period, the point at which the white blood cell, red blood cell, platelets, hemoglobin, and hematocrit laboratory values are at the lowest, the patient was treated with intravenous antibiotics and packed red blood cell and platelet transfusions. Seventeen days into his hospitalization, the patient developed a high-grade fever, spiking up to 103.2°F. The febrile period continued intermittently for the next 5 days. The patient became bed-bound because of the debilitating side effects of the chemotherapy regimen and accompanying infection. On the morning of day 22, the patient had received premedications for an additional course of chemotherapy, which included a benzodiazepine. As the patient was getting up to use the urinal, he lost his balance, falling forward and hitting his head on the counter across from his bed. The patient's wife was present in the room at the time of the fall. Before his fall, his Johns Hopkins Fall Assessment Score was 8 or Moderate Risk. The physician was immediately notified and a stat CT of the head was performed. The patient's platelet count was 12,000/mm³ at the time of the fall. The patient did develop a bruise on his forehead. The CT was negative for a subdural hematoma.

The case study illustrates findings from the quality improvement project. A combination of factors, including debilitation and medication, contributed to the fall.

Table 1	
Mean laboratory values	
Laboratory Test	**Mean Laboratory Value**
Red blood cell count	3.25 million cells/μL
Platelet count	139,000/μL (range: 7000–328,000/μL)
Hemoglobin	9.6 g/dL
Hematocrit	29%

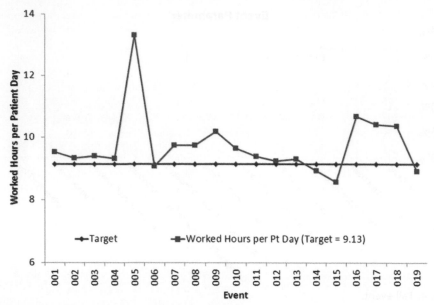

Fig. 5. Worked hours per patient day.

Although thrombocytopenia is not a contributing factor to the fall, a low platelet count can significantly impact the extent of a patient's injury.

After completion of the initial data review, the hospital implemented the use of yellow nonskid socks and yellow armbands to easily identify patients at risk for falls. In September 2011, staff meetings/in-services were held to outline and describe the various components of the Johns Hopkins Hospital Fall Assessment tool. During the sessions, purposeful rounding was reemphasized (**Fig. 6**). Additional discussion included the impact of medications (such as narcotics, antihypertensives, and

The 5 P's

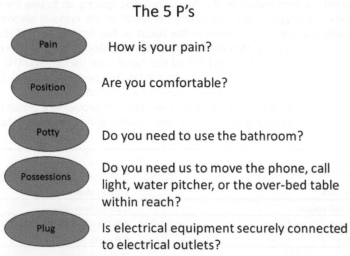

Pain	How is your pain?
Position	Are you comfortable?
Potty	Do you need to use the bathroom?
Possessions	Do you need us to move the phone, call light, water pitcher, or the over-bed table within reach?
Plug	Is electrical equipment securely connected to electrical outlets?

Fig. 6. Purposeful rounding.

diuretics) on falls and fall risk. Staff also reviewed interventions to address fall prevention in the areas of low, moderate, and high risk. With the assistance of the Quality Director, the unit was able to determine the fall per 1000-patient-day rate on a monthly basis. These initial steps led to a slight decrease in falls (**Fig. 7**).

Shortly after completion of the project, the oncology units relocated within the hospital campus to an existing building that had been renovated. A few months after the move, a fall team led by the weekend supervisor debuted. The team implemented a back-to-basics approach to fall prevention. Baseline knowledge was evaluated. Staff received additional education on identifying at-risk patients and was revalidated on use of the bed alarm system. A patient-focused S.A.F.E. tool was adapted from a hospital within the health care system. The tool emphasizes issues unique to the oncology population (**Fig. 8**). The fall team meets every 2 months and reviews all unit falls for opportunities for improvement. A patient member was added to the team. The interventions have decreased falls with injury, which are currently less than the NDNQI mean. Fall reduction remains a challenge.

IMPLICATION FOR PRACTICE

In the oncology population, disease process and treatment factors place patients at risk for falls. Patients with hematologic disease are at risk as a direct result of the disease process or treatment. Low red blood cell count and hemoglobin/hematocrit can contribute to feelings of fatigue and dizziness. Patients with metastatic disease to the brain and bone may be at increased risk because of cognitive issues and the potential for pathologic fracture. Thrombocytopenia (disease-related or treatment-induced) increases risk of injuries associated with falls.

Fall bundles provide a framework for developing comprehensive fall programs for oncology units. A change in unit or hospital culture may be necessary before program implementation. Consistent hourly rounding is one program element that is easy to implement and can provide immediate impact.

Interventional studies in the oncology population have focused on education and increased mobility. Small sample size and focus on ambulatory and geriatric populations limit the applicability of results. Interventions unique to populations, such as

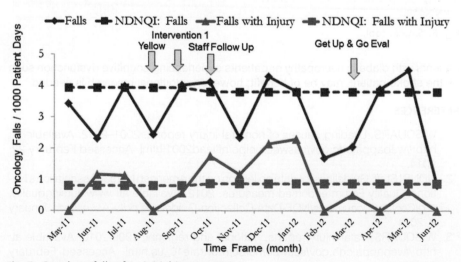

Fig. 7. Oncology falls after initial interventions.

KEEPING YOU S.A.F.E.

Your safety and well-being is our primary goal. Our aim is to reduce the risk for potential problems while you are receiving treatment. One of the potential problems is falls. We want to make sure that you are safe while you are at our facility. Our S.A.F.E slogan is a simple reminder for you and our staff to:

S - make sure that your **SURROUNDING** is clear

A - **ASK** for help, especially if you feel weak or dizzy

F - involve your **FAMILY** or **FRIENDS**

E - **EDUCATE** the patient and family regarding safety

KEEPING OUR PATIENTS "SAFE" IS PART OF OUR CARE.

It is important for you to know that:

- Some patients feel weak and fatigued (tired) after receiving chemotherapy.
- Certain medications may have some side effects, such as lowering your blood pressure, dizziness, and feeling weak when you get up from lying down.
- When you receive medications that may cause dizziness or sleepiness, your bed alarm will be turned on for four (4) hours for your safety.
- There are several pieces of equipment around you that you do not normally have, such as IV pump and poles, cords, tubes, and so on. Having these around may increase your risk for fall.
- Please do not push buttons or turn off the alarm on your IV.
  Please do not turn off the bed alarms.
- If you have a family member or a friend in the room and you need to go to the bathroom, call the nurse for help. Although a friend or family member can learn to help, we want to make sure that you are safe. Your friend or family member can learn from the nurse how to assist you safely when you are home.
- Use the call light to call for assistance at anytime.
- Keep the yellow non-slip socks on at all times.

REMEMBER:

Always ask for help before getting out of bed or chair when you feel unsteady or weak.

Platelets are responsible for clotting. A fall with low platelets can be fatal!

I have been instructed on keeping myself safe.	
NAME:_____	Room:_____
CAREGIVER:_____	
RN NAME:_____	Date:_____

Fig. 8. S.A.F.E. tool.

patients with diabetic neuropathy or patients experiencing cognitive dysfunction such as the stroke patient, may be of benefit; however, additional research is needed.

REFERENCES

1. WISQUARS. Leading causes of nonfatal injury reports. 2001–2012. Available at: http://webappa.cdc.gov/sasweb/ncipc/nfilead2001.html. Accessed February 22, 2014.
2. NDNQI Staff. Guidelines for data collection on the American Nurses Association's National Quality Forum endorsed measures. 2012. Available at: www.nursingquality.org/Content/Documents/NQF-Data-Collection-Guidelines.pdf. Accessed January 2, 2014.
3. WISQUARS. Fatal injury reports, national and regional, 1999-2010. Available at: http://webappa.cdc.gov/sasweb/ncipc/mortrate10_us.html. Accessed February 22, 2014.

4. Ang E, Mordiffi S, Wong H. Evaluating the use of a targeted multiple intervention strategy in reducing patient falls in an acute care hospital: a randomized controlled trial. J Adv Nurs 2011;67(9):1984–92.
5. Bonuel N, Manjos A, Lockett L, et al. Best practice fall prevention strategies. Crit Care Nurs Q 2011;9:154–8.
6. Boushon B, Nielsen G, Quigley P, et al. How-to guide: reducing patient injuries from falls. 2012. Available at: www.ihi.org. Accessed January 2, 2014.
7. Agency for Healthcare Research and Quality. Preventing falls in hospitals: a toolkit for improving quality of care. Available at: http://www.ahrq.gov/professionals/systems/hospital/fallpxtoolkit/fallpxtoolkit.pdf. Accessed February 22, 2014.
8. Titler M, Shever L, Kanak M, et al. Factors associated with falls during hospitalization in an older adult population. Res Theory Nurs Pract 2011;25(5):127–52.
9. Lew F, Qu X. Effects of multi-joint muscular fatigue on biomechanics of slips. J Biomech 2014;47(1):59–64.
10. Miller L, Limbaugh C. Applying evidence to develop a medical oncology fall-prevention program. Clin J Oncol Nurs 2008;12(1):158–60.
11. Olrich T, Kallman M, Nigolian C. Hourly rounding: a replication study. Medsurg Nurs 2012;21(1):23–6, 36.
12. Yates K, Tart R. Acute care patient falls: evaluation of a revised fall prevention program following comparative analysis of psychiatric and medical patient falls. Appl Nurs Res 2012;25:68–74.
13. Allan-Gibbs R. Falls and hospitalized patients with cancer: a review of the literature. Clin J Oncol Nurs 2010;14(6):784–92.
14. Spoelstra S, Given B, Given W. Fall prevention in hospitals: an integrative review. Clin Nurs Res 2012;21:92–112.
15. Anderson O, Boshier P, Hanna G. Interventions designed to prevent healthcare bed-related injuries in patients [review]. Cochrane Database Syst Rev 2012;3: 1–30.
16. Hardin S, Dienemann J, Rudisil P, et al. Inpatient fall prevention: use of in-room Webcams. J Patient Saf 2013;9:29–35.
17. Millman E, Pronovost P, Makary M, et al. Patient-assisted incident reporting: Including the patient in patient safety. J Patient Saf 2011;7(2):106–8.
18. Lloyd T. Creation of a multi-interventional fall-prevention program. Orthop Nurs 2011;30(4):249–57.
19. Stone C, Lawlor P, Savva G, et al. Prospective study of falls and risk factors for falls in adults with advanced cancer. J Clin Oncol 2012;30(17):2128–33.
20. Capone L, Albert N, Bena J, et al. Serious fall injuries in hospitalized patients with and without cancer. J Nurs Care Qual 2013;28(1):52–9.
21. Winters-Stone K, Torgrimson B, Horak F, et al. Identifying factors associated with falls in postmenopausal breast cancer survivors: a multi-disciplinary approach. Arch Phys Med Rehabil 2011;92:646–52.
22. Nabholtz JM. Long-term safety of aromatase inhibitors in the treatment of breast cancer. Ther Clin Risk Manag 2008;4(1):189–204.
23. Bylow K, Hemmerich J, Mohile S, et al. Obese frailty, physical performance deficits, and falls in older men with biochemical recurrence of prostate cancer on androgen deprivation therapy: a case-control study. Urology 2011;77(4): 934–40.
24. Overcash J, Beckstead J. Predicting falls in older patients using components of a comprehensive geriatric assessment. Clin J Oncol Nurs 2008;12(6):941–9.
25. Capone L, Albert M, Bena J, et al. Predictors of a fall event in hospitalized patients with cancer. Oncol Nurs Forum 2012;39(5):407–15.

26. Cozart HC, Cesario S. Falls aren't us. State of the science. Crit Care Nurs Q 2009; 32(2):116–27.

27. Tofthagen C, Visovsky C, Berry D. Strength and balance training for adults with peripheral neuropathy and high risk of fall: current evidence and implications for future research. Oncol Nurs Forum 2012;39(5):416–24.

28. McLaughlin T, Wittstein E, White T, et al. Moving to wellness. A pilot study examining a nurse-driven exercise program in acutely ill patients with cancer. Clin J Oncol Nurs 2012;16(3):105–10.

29. Potter P, Olsen S, Kuhrik M, et al. A DVD program on fall prevention skills training for cancer family caregivers. J Cancer Educ 2011;27:83–90.

Overview of Extracorporeal Membrane Oxygenation in Cardiogenic Shock

Dena Allen, MSN, RN, PhD(c), CCRN[a,*],
Barbara Leeper, MN, RN-BC, CNS M-S, CCRN[b]

KEYWORDS

- ECMO • Extracorporeal membrane oxygenation • Ventricular assist devices
- Cardiogenic shock • ECMO program development

KEY POINTS

- Patients with cardiovascular disease who are admitted to the cardiac care unit have higher case mix indexes and increased critical illness.
- Cardiogenic shock is associated with the development of a systemic inflammatory response syndrome contributing to hemodynamic instability.
- The use of extracorporeal membrane oxygenator (ECMO) support for cardiogenic shock is increasing due to the availability of smaller devices.
- An ECMO program can be successfully managed by experienced critical care nurses with advanced hemodynamic and oxygenation expertise.

In recent years, the use of extracorporeal membrane oxygenators (ECMO) has proliferated in cardiovascular intensive care units (ICUs) partially due to advances in technology with the development of smaller, more portable machines, but also owing to the increasing numbers of patients with end-stage heart failure and cardiogenic shock. Another contributing factor surfaced in 2009 with the H1N1 influenza outbreak and again recently in January and February 2014. A serious complication of the H1N1 influenza is acute respiratory failure with "white out" of the lungs on chest x-ray. The use of ECMO has been found to improve survival rates in this deadly situation. The purpose of this article was to discuss the transition of the cardiovascular ICU in the United States, review cardiogenic shock etiologies and the role of ECMO, and discuss the process of implementing a nurse-run ECMO program.

Disclosures: The authors have nothing to disclose.
[a] Coronary Care Unit, Baylor University Medical Center at Dallas, 3500 Gaston Avenue, Truett Building, Suite 145, Dallas, TX 75246, USA; [b] Cardiovascular Services, Baylor University Medical Center at Dallas, 3500 Gaston Avenue, Truett Building, Suite 145, Dallas, TX 75246, USA
* Corresponding author.
E-mail address: Dena.Allen@baylorhealth.edu

Crit Care Nurs Clin N Am 26 (2014) 581–588
http://dx.doi.org/10.1016/j.ccell.2014.08.002
0899-5885/14/$ – see front matter © 2014 Elsevier Inc. All rights reserved.

TRANSFORMATION OF THE CARDIOVASCULAR INTENSIVE CARE UNIT

The coronary care unit (CCU) has played a pivotal role in the management of patients with coronary artery disease. Over time, and since the opening of the first CCU, outcomes associated with the management of life-threatening rhythm disturbances and prompt recognition and management of acute myocardial infarction (AMI) have improved markedly. In recent years, it has become apparent that the landscape of the CCU has dramatically changed. Although survival rates after AMI have improved, the prevalence of other cardiovascular related diseases has also increased.[1] Katz and colleagues[1] examined temporal trends in patient characteristics, processes of care, and in-hospital outcomes among unselected admissions within todays CCU. Their findings confirmed significant changes have occurred. The number of ST-segment elevation myocardial infarction patients declined, and there has been an increase in the number of non-ST-segment elevation myocardial infarction patients. The volume of patients with noncardiovascular diagnoses, particularly with comorbid critical illnesses, including sepsis, acute kidney injury, and respiratory failure, has grown.[1] More patients are intubated with mechanical ventilator support and are on renal replacement therapy. These changes can be attributed to changing demographics of patients, including an increased volume of elderly, female, and minority patients.[2] The incidence of chronic illness has increased dramatically including diabetes, hypertension, renal insufficiency/failure, and chronic obstructive pulmonary disease. These conditions are now present in many patients with cardiovascular disease admitted to the CCU today. The final result is higher case mix indexes and increased critical illness.[2]

Recently, there has been an escalation of the number of patients being admitted to the cardiovascular ICU with acute and/or end-stage heart failure. These patients are often in cardiogenic shock. Various pharmacologic interventions (inotropes and vasoactive infusions) are initiated along with the insertion of mechanical assist devices, including an intraaortic balloon pump and ventricular assist devices (either percutaneous or implantable), to stabilize these patients. When these interventions are ineffective, patients are often placed on ECMO. These patients often develop multisystem organ dysfunction requiring extensive resources. Morrow and colleagues[2] described some large centers having developed specialized "heart failure ICUs" for the purpose of caring for this patient population.

CARDIOGENIC SHOCK AND MECHANICAL CIRCULATORY SUPPORT
Cardiogenic Shock

Cardiogenic shock is defined as having a cardiac index of 2.2 L/min^2 or less with evidence of tissue hypoperfusion. Associated findings include hypotension, delayed capillary refill, decreased urine output, decreased level of consciousness, and cool and mottled extremities. The most common cause of cardiogenic shock is AMI with an associated loss of 45% to 50% of viable myocardium. It may also occur when there is a mechanical complication of AMI, such as acute mitral regurgitation or a perforated intraventricular septum. The other most common causes are those patients with acute decompensated heart failure and end-stage cardiomyopathy. **Box 1** provides a list of etiologies for cardiogenic shock.[3] Individuals found to be at greatest risk for development of cardiogenic shock include those who are older, female, diabetic, have had an anterior MI or history of previous MI, reduced ejection fraction, or larger MI evidenced by higher cardiac enzyme levels. Patients with a history of peripheral vascular disease or prior cerebrovascular accident also have an increased risk.[3]

> **Box 1**
> **Etiologies of cardiogenic shock**
>
> - AMI
> - Mechanical complications of AMI
>   - Acute mitral valve regurgitation
>   - Perforated Intraventricular septum
> - Post pump cardiogenic shock after cardiopulmonary bypass
> - Isolated right ventricular failure
> - Cardiac tamponade
> - Myocarditis
> - Acute decompensated heart failure
> - End-stage cardiomyopathy
> - Valvular heart disease
>
> *Abbreviation:* AMI, acute myocardial infarction.
> *Data from* Josephson L. Cardiogenic shock. Dimens Crit Care Nurs 2008;27(4):160–70; and Tuggle D. Optimizing hemodynamics: strategies for fluid and medication titration in shock. In: Carlson KK, editor. AACN advanced critical care nursing. St Louis (MO): Saunders Elsevier; 2009. p. 1099–133.

After an AMI, there may be myocardial tissue that is stunned or hibernating. Stunned myocardium refers to tissue that does not function normally after an ischemic event despite restoration of normal blood flow. Hibernating myocardium occurs when there is a chronic reduction in perfusion to an area of muscle. The cells adapt to the reduction of blood flow by downregulating oxygen demands. Once perfusion is restored, the involved tissue returns to normal.[3]

Loss of viable myocardium may not account for the sole cause of cardiogenic shock. There is evidence suggesting cardiogenic shock is associated with the development of a systemic inflammatory response syndrome contributing to hemodynamic instability.[4] Patients exhibit increased body temperature, elevated white blood cell counts, complement, interleukins, C-reactive protein, and other proinflammatory biomarkers. Nitric oxide, a potent vasodilator that is normally cardioprotective, is released by many cells, reaching toxic levels, and has many deleterious effects.[5] This contributes to the continuation of the inflammatory response and further myocardial depression.

Mechanical Circulatory Support

Over the past 2 decades, mechanical circulatory support has contributed to more aggressive interventions for cardiogenic shock. The purpose of mechanical circulatory support is to "restore cardiac output and preserve end-organ perfusion, off-load the left ventricle, optimize the balance between oxygen supply and demand, and allow for recovery of ischemic but viable myocardium."[4] There are many devices, including the intraaortic balloon pump, percutaneous and implantable mechanical assist devices, and ECMO, available to the clinician.

The mainstay of the management of cardiogenic shock has been the intraaortic balloon pump. However, if the patient demonstrates inadequate tissue oxygen delivery despite pharmacologic interventions as well as intraaortic balloon pump, then advanced circulatory support should be considered. ECMO was first used in adults in 1972.[6] Since then, there have been several reports of ECMO being used to manage cardiogenic shock. The Extracorporeal Life Support Organization has a registry for those ECMO centers who participate. The number of ECMO cases for cardiogenic shock in adults dramatically increased in 2009 and has continued to grow. Survival rates to discharge vary slightly but the Extracorporeal Life Support Organization notes that the cumulative rate is approximately 45% to 50%.[7] Individual groups report survival rates in the cardiac failure population to be 33%.[8] Smedira and colleagues[9] investigated 5-year survival rates after ECMO for cardiac failure patients, assessed survival after bridge to transplant or weaning from ECMO, and identified factors influencing the outcomes. Two hundred adult patients were enrolled in their study. Survival at 3 days was 76%, at 30 days was 38%, and at 5 years was 24%. Those patients who were surviving at 30 days had a 63% chance of 5-year survival. Forty-eight percent of these patients underwent a heart transplant and 71 were weaned from ECMO with the intent of survival. Survival rates at 5 years for these 2 groups was 44% and 40%, respectively.

ECMO is similar to cardiopulmonary bypass where venous blood is removed from the body via a large central vein, pumped through an oxygenator, and then returned to the arterial circulation via a cannula in a large artery. The oxygenator consists of small hollow fibers allowing the exchange of oxygen and carbon dioxide. Blood flow is maintained by a centrifugal pump that is able to deliver high flow rates with little trauma to the blood cells. Peripheral access as described above is easier to achieve but other access points can be used as well. There are 2 types of ECMO, venovenous and venoarterial. Patients in cardiogenic shock will have venoarterial ECMO unless complicated by the onset of respiratory failure, which is an indication for venovenous ECMO (**Fig. 1**). Venoarterial ECMO has been identified as the fastest growing indication for ECMO worldwide.[6]

Complications

ECMO can present many challenges for our patients. Complications include limb ischemia, hemorrhage, pulmonary edema, and thromboembolism.[4] These patients are at high risk for infection either through the cannulation sites or when accessing the lines for blood gas measurements. Meticulous aseptic technique must be used, as for any central line. The failing ventricle may dilate, contributing to worsening failure. Frequent echocardiography is recommended to monitor for this situation. If it occurs, the cannulation sites may need to be changed to a more central location.[6] Another challenge is the length of time a patient may be on ECMO. The duration of support is limited based on the patient's status and tolerance, as well as recovery or need for other devices or transplant.

THE DEVELOPMENT OF AN EXTRACORPOREAL MEMBRANE OXYGENATION PROGRAM

In July of 2012, we abruptly admitted our first 2 patients on ECMO to our cardiovascular ICU. One was on ECMO as a bridge to transplantation and the other was a bridge to another ventricular assist device. Our nursing staff provided care for the patients and the perfusionist remained at the bedside to care for the ECMO circuit. Initially, this was an exciting venture; however, we soon realized that this was only the beginning of a long-term commitment. We began to admit several more patients on ECMO, most with cardiogenic shock associated with end-stage cardiomyopathies or after AMI. The nursing staff quickly realized more formal education was required. The

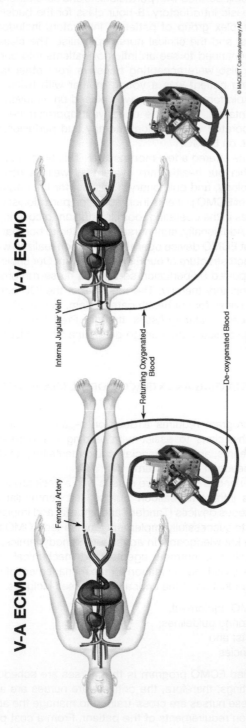

Fig. 1. Examples of the cannulation sites for venoarterial ECMO (femoral vein–femoral artery) and venovenous ECMO (femoral vein–internal jugular vein) with blood flow through the oxygenator. (Used with permission from MAQUET Cardiopulmonary AG, Rasttat, Germany.)

clinical nurse specialist collaborated with perfusionists and cardiothoracic surgeons to develop content for a basic introductory, 8-hour class for the bedside nursing staff caring for this very complex group of patients. Instructors included perfusionists, cardiothoracic surgeons, and the clinical nurse specialist. The class was taught in September 2012. We continued to see an influx of patients into our unit on ECMO on a routine basis. We also were accepting transfers from other facilities in North Texas. Our most exciting patient was a young mother with twins who had cystic fibrosis and chronic respiratory failure. She was placed on venovenous ECMO as a bridge to lung transplantation, which she underwent approximately 6 weeks later. The nursing staff collaborated with physical therapy and perfusionists to ambulate her in the hall daily while on ECMO.

An additional class was offered a few months later. This time, there were requests from other entities within our health care system as well as other service lines, including trauma, cardiology, and pulmonary medicine, for their adult cystic fibrosis patients. As the volume of ECMO patients increased, the perfusionists were struggling with trying to cover cases in the operating room in addition to covering the patients in the cardiovascular ICU. Additionally, staff nurses continued to bombard the perfusionists with questions about ECMO device operation. We soon realized we had to make a decision about the support structure of our ECMO program. Our choices were to have a program run and supported by perfusion services, a nurse-run program, or a program supported by respiratory therapy. The manager of the ICU consulted with the Director of Perfusion Services for our health care system, the Chief of Cardiac Transplantation and Mechanical Circulatory Assist, the Vice President of Critical Care Services, and the rest of the clinical care team to determine which discipline would lead the new ECMO program.

CONSIDERATIONS FOR STARTING AN EXTRACORPOREAL MEMBRANE OXYGENATION PROGRAM

Beginning an ECMO program requires a decision regarding which discipline will collaborate with the physicians to assist with leading the program. The clinical strength, tenure of the teams, and the financial requirements help to determine which discipline best fits the needs of the program.

The utilization of experienced critical care nurses with a back ground in mechanical assist devices such as intraaortic balloon pumps, left ventricular assist devices, including both percutaneous devices (Tandem and Impella) and implantable ventricular assist devices helps to successfully implement a nurse-led ECMO program. These experienced nurses are knowledgeable in advanced hemodynamics, critical titration of vasopressors, vasodilators, inotropic agents, and mechanical ventilation. Their advanced clinical skills support the foundation for the management of the ECMO technology. The additional education of the critical care nurses includes:

- Review of the ECMO equipment;
- Patient care monitoring guidelines;
- Safety requirements; and
- Managing emergencies.

A benefit of a nurse-led ECMO program is that nurses are scheduled around the clock in acute care settings; therefore, the critical care nurses are always available if ECMO is initiated. These nurses are cross-trained to manage the advanced hemodynamic and oxygenation requirements of the patient. From a cost perspective, this model allows for more efficient use of the nursing staff and their advanced skill set.

A perfusionist-led program requires the perfusionist to remain at the bedside for 24 hours a day, as long as the ECMO patient remains in the ICU. The perfusionists have had formal training and are experts in ECMO technology. They are able to prime the lines, assist with emergency insertions, troubleshoot the circuit, and discontinue the device. Depending on the program, perfusionists may be employees of the hospital or may be part of a contract agency. Having consistent perfusionists is essential in developing an ECMO program. The challenge with this model is related to the coverage the perfusionists have to provide, not only for the ECMO patient, but also for covering cases in the operating room. A high ECMO case volume can contribute to burnout to the perfusionists fairly quickly.

The potential cost implications must be considered with this model. If the perfusionist is employed by the facility or their services are contracted, this cost can significantly impact the overall cost of the program. There is a savings of approximately $30,000 per patient when a nurse-led program is in place compared with a perfusionist-led program. Perfusionist costs are not individually reimbursable and are part of a diagnosis-related group for the ECMO case. This cost savings can make a tremendous impact on the bottom line at a time most hospitals are striving to meet Medicare reimbursement rates.

In a respiratory therapist-led ECMO program, the therapists are usually registered respiratory therapists. The therapists learn mechanical ventilation and gas exchange concepts in their formal training programs. ECMO technology utilizes both concepts and this knowledge is essential in implementing a successful program. Registered respiratory therapists must have additional training in advanced hemodynamic monitoring, knowledge of vasoactive medications, and orientation to the ECMO equipment.

A registered respiratory therapist–led program can also lead to substantial cost savings. The cost savings for cardiac and pulmonary ECMO patients would be approximately $16,000 and $23,000, respectively. This decision may be driven by the availability of registered respiratory therapists in a given community and is a determining factor in the type of ECMO program implemented.

All 3 ECMO-led program options may be effective for an acute care setting hospital. Specific program needs and resource availability determine which program is selected. We made the decision to collaborate with perfusion services to develop a nurse-run ECMO program at Baylor University Medical Center. The manager identified the most experienced nurses with advanced hemodynamic and oxygenation skills from day and night shifts. These nurses were asked to commit to being available to being on call whenever an ECMO patient was being admitted including 24 hours per day, 7 days a week. Nine RNs volunteered to commit to the program. These 9 nurses became our ECMO nurse specialists within a few months.

The perfusionists began to hold wet labs weekly for these 9 individuals. Each nurse attended these for 6 weeks for focused training and ECMO competency testing. The wet labs lasted approximately 2 hours each. These nurses were precepted by a perfusionist at the bedside. The perfusionist shared didactic information and hands-on experience during the precepted shifts. Troubleshooting the circuit was essential for emergency situations. The ECMO specialists requested to attend a training program at a nationally recognized site. Upon their return, they commented that the course they attended reinforced what they had already learned. These 9 nurses helped to create the initial nurse-led program.

Gradually, the nursing team started to prepare and assist the perfusionist with ECMO insertion. The nurse-led program was promoted and nurses were challenged to learn more in their new roles because of limited perfusionist availability.

Perfusionists are required to prime the system as well as to attach the continuous renal replacement therapy cannulae to the ECMO system.

Eighteen months later, this ECMO program has been successful in our institution. There have been no adverse events in our nurse-led program. This initiative has contributed to increased retention of our nursing staff who have participated in the challenge of running this program. We have positive feedback from patients and their families when they come back to thank the staff for their compassion and care during their stay. Today, we are a referral center for complicated cardiac and pulmonary compromised patients.

SUMMARY

This is an example of a process employed by our leadership and nursing staff to implement the use of ECMO support for a very high-risk patient population. Our success can be attributed to the engagement of all members of the team to support and promote the contributions of the tenured bedside nursing staff to build this ECMO program. We are continuing to see an influx of patients on ECMO owing to a variety of conditions in our cardiovascular ICU. The overall program has contributed to the satisfaction of everyone who has participated in the growth of the program.

REFERENCES

1. Katz JN, Shah BR, Volz EM, et al. Evolution of the coronary care unit: clinical characteristics and temporal trends in healthcare delivery and outcomes. Crit Care Med 2010;38(2):375–81.
2. Morrow DA, Fang JC, Fintel DJ, et al. Evolution of critical care cardiology: transformation of the cardiovascular intensive care unit and the emerging need for new medical staffing and training models: a Scientific statement from the American Heart Association. Circulation 2012;126:1408–28.
3. McAtee ME. Cardiogenic shock. Crit Care Nurs Clin North Am 2011;23(4): 6-7-615.
4. Abu-Omar Y, Tsui SS. Mechanical circulatory support for AMI and cardiogenic shock. J Cardiovasc Surg 2010;25:434–41.
5. Hochman JS. Cardiogenic shock complicating acute myocardial infarction: expanding the paradigm. Circulation 2003;107:2998–3002.
6. Cove ME, MacLaren G. Clinical review: mechanical circulatory support for cardiogenic shock complicating acute myocardial infarction. Crit Care 2010;14:235–46.
7. Conrad SA, Rycus PT. The registry of the extracorporeal life support organization. In: Annich GM, Lynch WR, MacLaren G, et al, editors. ECMO extracorporeal cardiopulmonary support in critical care, 4th edition. Ann Arbor (MI): Extracorporeal Life Support Organization; 2012. p. 87–104.
8. Marasco SF, Lukas G, McDonald M, et al. Review of ECMO (extra corporeal membrane oxygenation) support in critically ill adult patients. Heart Lung Circ 2008; 17S:S41–7.
9. Smedira NG, Moazami N, Golding CM, et al. Clinical experience with 202 adults receiving extracorporeal membrane oxygenation for cardiac failure: survival at five years. J Thorac Cardiovasc Surg 2001;122(1):92–102.

Transitional Care Models

Preventing Readmissions for High-Risk Patient Populations

Mae M. Centeno, DNP, RN, CCNS, ACNS-BC[a],*,
Kellie L. Kahveci, MSN, RN, AGPCNP-BC, GNP-BC, CHFN[b]

KEYWORDS

- Readmissions • Transitional care • Elderly • Geriatric

KEY POINTS

- Factors influencing need for hospital readmission reduction programs are identified.
- Initial transitional care program outcomes are described.
- Modifications made to transitional care program based on barriers identified are discussed.
- Lessons learned and recommendations for future programs are identified.

Chronic illness is a significant problem in the United States. Approximately 80% of older adults have 1 chronic condition, and 50% have at least 2.[1] Among chronic conditions, heart failure and pneumonia occur most frequently. In 2010, patients aged 65 years and older accounted for 69% of heart failure hospitalizations.[2] Specific data related to pneumonia are less available; however, this condition is targeted by the Centers for Medicare & Medicaid (CMS).[3]

Approximately 20% of Medicare patients are readmitted within 30 days of hospital discharge. In October 2012, the CMS began penalizing hospitals for excessive readmission rates related to hospital discharges for heart failure, pneumonia, and acute myocardial infarction.[3] This article shares the experience of a large metropolitan health care system working to decrease readmission rates for this patient population using a transitional care program.

Disclosure: The authors have no disclosures to report.
a Chronic Care Continuum, Institute of Chronic Disease and Care Redesign, Baylor Health Care System at Dallas, 8080 North Central Expressway, Dallas, TX 75206, USA; b Baylor HouseCalls and Transitional Care Program, Health Texas Provider Network, 4004 Worth Street Suite 200, Dallas, TX 75246, USA
* Corresponding author.
E-mail address: Mae.Centeno@baylorhealth.edu

Crit Care Nurs Clin N Am 26 (2014) 589–597
http://dx.doi.org/10.1016/j.ccell.2014.08.009
0899-5885/14/$ – see front matter © 2014 Elsevier Inc. All rights reserved.

TRANSITIONAL CARE PILOT

A large metropolitan hospital system in the Southwestern United States began efforts focused in the inpatient setting, which improved readmission rates for patients with acute myocardial infarction but not with heart failure or pneumonia. Studies have shown improvement in readmission rates through transitional care interventions and coordination of care.[4,5] The system developed a team to begin work to improve patient care, thereby decreasing rehospitalization rates. The team initially targeted heart failure. The transitional care model described by Naylor and colleagues[4] was the model of care chosen.

The transitional care team was integrated into the system's well-established primary care house calls program. This practice provided the new program with existing infrastructure and in-home expertise that would not have been afforded had the program started in isolation.

The transitional care model was piloted in one of the system's suburban community hospitals. The goal of the transitional care pilot program was to decrease readmission rates for patients aged 65 years and older with heart failure. A team was assembled that included social work and care coordination, administration, nursing, and physician leadership. A nurse practitioner (NP), an employee of the practice management arm of the health care system, and the medical director were contracted and credentialed by the hospital. The NP collaborated with the social worker and care coordinator to identify patients meeting program criteria. Potential patients were identified using work lists, which included diagnostic-related group codes, elevated brain natriuretic peptide levels, and the prescription of intravenous diuretics.

After patients were identified as potential program candidates, a physician's order was required for transitional care and geriatric consult. For patients admitted with a diagnosis of heart failure, the order was included in the standardized heart failure order set. After order receipt, the NP reviewed the chart to ensure inclusion criteria were met, and then discussed the program with the patient and/or surrogate decision maker, performed geriatric assessment, and received consent to see the patient in their home. A note was written in the medical record documenting the consult and the patient's transitional care status.

Inclusion criteria included residing within 15 miles of target hospital, individuals aged 65 years or older, primary diagnosis of heart failure, and returning home, defined as a private residence, assisted living facility, or residential care home. In contrast to the work of Naylor and colleagues,[4] the program included patients with significant cognitive deficits and those without phones. Patients who would be receiving hospice care, had end-stage renal disease, and were homeless were not initially excluded; however, after the team attempted unsuccessfully to follow patients with these additional characteristics, the criteria were modified to exclude them. **Box 1** lists the protocol.

The pilot program reduced 30-day readmission rates by 48%; however, the costs of the program were high.[6] The team began discussing methods to maintain the achievements that resulted in decreased hospital readmission, while simultaneously targeting costs and possible overuse of resources. Before expanding the transitional care program to other facilities, consideration was given to several issues, and modifications were integrated into the model.

In the pilot, 4 barriers to appropriate care and potential cost savings were identified by the team. Identification of appropriate patients was problematic; nearly as many patients with heart failure as those without were followed in their homes. Some of the patients followed by the NP did not seem to require such intense intervention. If

Box 1
Transitional care protocol followed by NPs
Visit patients in the acute care setting on order receipt and daily as indicated
Initial in-home visit within 48 hours of hospital discharge on regular business days
Conduct visits every week for 4 weeks and every other week for an additional 8 weeks, with as-needed visits if a change in condition occurs; on call for assistance 24/7
Educate patients and family members on disease process, medications, and self-care management
Document goals of care, including advance care planning
Diagnosis and treat other acute conditions as needed
Order and coordination of home health and hospice services and durable medical equipment
Titration of heart failure medications
Collaboration with hospital-based social workers for NP-identified social issues
Engagement of community pharmacists to assist with unique medication problems
Attend visits with patient to primary care physician/cardiologist.
Coordinate care with the primary care physician during the patient's time in transitional care

risk could be stratified and other less costly interventions substituted, expenses could potentially be decreased. There was significant need for a role other than that of the NP to collect data and assume responsibility for reporting. The NPs suggested that they were not the best qualified to meet some of the patients needs; specifically, social work and pharmacologic expertise were identified as areas of need. Finally, the team suggested a Master's-prepared nurse, such as the NP, was not needed for some of the care delivered.

APPROPRIATE PATIENT IDENTIFICATION AND PREDICTING RISK OF READMISSION

With finite resources, predictive modeling may help clinicians design interventions to best meet patient needs. Health care systems have begun to address issues of patient identification and risk stratification.

Amarasingham and colleagues[7] designed and implemented automated risk modeling software that accurately identifies patients at high risk for readmission or death in real-time. The model includes data extracted from an electronic medical record, including physiologic, laboratory, demographic, and utilization variables within 24 hours of hospital admission. The patients are then placed into risk categories. A compiled list is accessible to clinicians and case managers, notifying them of patients at highest risk. This predictive modeling reduced the Medicare heart failure readmissions by 33%.

The Preventable Admissions Care Team (PACT) at The Mount Sinai Medical Center in New York used admission history data to identify and target for intervention patients at high risk for readmission. The team was able to validate that hospitalization history alone is a reasonable proxy for more formal multivariable regression models in predicting 30-day readmission risk, allowing them to implement interventions based on risk. The psychosocial drivers of readmission are assessed and addressed through a 35-day social work–led intervention that begins on discharge. Through this personalized follow-up care, PACT has been successful in reducing 30-day readmissions by 56% and emergency department visits by 51% for high-risk patients.[8]

In the transitional care model described earlier, 14 clinical variables were required to calculate the predicted risk score of readmission. Although the information was available in the electronic health record, the tool required manual input of data by the NPs. After several months, the team noted that the tool did not discern patients at low risk of readmission.

Secondary to the challenges described, a decision was made to purchase Pulse 360, an application integrated into the electronic health record using patent-pending text and data aggregation to glean actionable information from available data to identify and risk stratify patient populations. The application analyzes and maps standard clinical notes and data in real time to quantitatively provide information on patients at risk for readmission, including the clinical and social variables contributing to the risk. The output is user-friendly and allows for communication and coordination within the application among team members.[9]

In the transitional care model described, the team follows 3 levels of risk. High-risk patients are offered in-home NP visits per protocol and Tel-Assurance (described later); moderate-risk patients are offered Tel-Assurance and scripted, protocol-based calls by the team RN at 3, 7, 21 days; and as-needed and low-risk patients are offered Tel-Assurance. All patients have access to any team member during their transition period.

The team designed and has implemented protocols to escalate the level of intervention patients receives if their health status declines. The change in level of intervention may be made either urgently, in the case of rapid decline, or team members may present the proposed change for consideration at weekly team meetings. If team consensus is achieved, the level of intervention is adjusted accordingly.

REMOTE MONITORING

Myriad challenges face clinicians managing patients with chronic disease, including monitoring changes in symptoms and status, medication and dietary adherence, and behaviors to improve self-care management. Many studies have focused on strategies for telephone coaching and telemonitoring, revealing mixed results. Telephone health coaching generally involves regular phone calls between providers and patients, designed to offer support, answer questions, encourage healthy behaviors, and promote adherence to the plan of care. Telemonitoring involves the transfer of physiologic data, such as blood pressure, weight, electrocardiographic signals, and oxygen saturation levels through technology such as telephone lines or wireless networks. Similar to structured telephone support, this strategy may remove some of the geographic or funding barriers that limit in-home visits.[10]

Inglis and colleagues[10] reviewed structured telephone support and telemonitoring trials and found that telemonitoring reduced both mortality and heart failure–related hospitalizations. However, although the structured telephone support reduced heart failure–related hospitalization, no affect on mortality was noted.

Researchers in England retrospectively assessed outcomes in patients enrolled in regular telephone health coaching programs delivered by nurses. They found significant increases in emergency admissions and outpatient visits in those who received coaching compared with matched controls.[11]

Tel-Assurance, an interactive voice recognition and Web-based platform developed and validated by physicians and clinicians to monitor behavioral change remotely, was selected as the tool to assist the clinical team in coordinating the care of identified patients. Patients in the Tel-Assurance program place a phone call or log in to a remote patient monitoring system on a daily basis to report how they are feeling that day and whether they are experiencing any symptoms. Patient health is tracked by a clinical team, and variances are shared with care providers so that adjustments can be made in follow-up, medications, or dietary intake. Patients also receive daily health tips that help them understand their condition so they can make better lifestyle decisions.[12]

In the transitional care model described, these trends and variances are monitored daily by the office-based clinical team. Protocols have been developed and implemented to guide the team in contacting patients and caregivers and discussing patient status. Office-based team members may advise patients/caregivers directly or may collaborate with or refer patients to the responsible NP or to their primary care provider.

EXPANSION OF THE TRANSITIONAL CARE MODEL TEAM
Role of the Social Worker

Clinically, making an argument for the expertise of social work and pharmacy support is intuitive. The argument is more challenging in a primarily fee-for-service environment where these services are generally not reimbursable. The literature supports models making a positive impact on outcomes for the populations they serve.

Psychosocial issues such as limited health literacy, lack of self-management skills, unmet functional needs, lack of social support, and living alone have all been associated with adverse outcomes, including readmission and mortality.[13,14] These factors may help to explain high levels of nonadherence to outpatient medical follow-up visits. Jencks and colleagues[15] found that 50% of medical readmissions did not have an outpatient bill between hospital stays, which suggests that facilitating prompt outpatient follow-up visits may be important in preventing poor outcomes.

Social workers at Rush University Medical Center[16] have worked to bolster transitions between the acute and post-acute care settings in Illinois. The interventions are specifically designed to address psychosocial issues or inadequate access to community services, such as transportation, homemaker, and social support services. Targeting these elements in at-risk older adults could impact adherence to the plan of care and reduce the likelihood of adverse events.

The Enhanced Discharge Planning Program was designed at Rush to augment the inpatient hospital discharge planning practice. The program began as a pilot to address concerns reported by hospital discharge planning staff that older adults were especially vulnerable to adverse postdischarge outcomes. The Enhanced Discharge Planning Program was developed as a telephone-based intervention implemented by Master's-prepared social workers with experience in geriatrics and community-based practice to address needs beyond the scope and purpose of the acute hospital discharge planning process. More broadly, Rush was a founding member of The Illinois Transitional Care Consortium, a group of organizations that work together to develop and implement Bridge, a social work–led, interdisciplinary model of transitional care. Bridge social workers work with patients and caregivers after discharge to recognize gaps in care and intervene to resolve identified needs.[16]

The social worker in the transitional care model contacts all high-risk patients and reviews level of function, caregiver status, mobility, socioeconomics, and community-based resource needs. Interventions are made based on information ascertained. The social worker is an integral team member and makes significant contributions, meeting needs the NPs felt they met inadequately or not at all in the original model. Moderate- and low-risk patients have access to the social worker when needs are identified through variance in the telemonitoring system.

Role of the Pharmacist

Patients are frequently discharged from the hospital with changes to their medication regimens, and therefore medication discrepancies, nonadherence, and adverse drug events are common during transitions of care. Taylor Haynes and colleagues[17] found pharmacist-directed medication reconciliation to be time-consuming but the most important intervention in improving outcomes during transitions in care. The pharmacist was able to correct errors and provide medication counseling to study participants.

The pharmacist in the transitional care model plays a significant role in managing the medication reconciliation process to reduce errors, recognize drug-to-drug interactions, identify polypharmacy, and evaluate for efficacy and cost-effectiveness of medications prescribed. Additional benefits of adding pharmacy expertise include coaching patients and caregivers in safe drug use and the importance of medication adherence. The pharmacist has been invaluable in working with individuals with low levels of general and health literacy to devise realistic medication regimens, and in developing educational tools to facilitate adherence.

The pharmacist contacts all high-risk patients for medication reconciliation, coaching, and counseling. Moderate- and low-risk patients are contacted based on discrepancies in the medication list and variance in the telemonitoring system.

Role of the Registered Nurse

Registered nurses are an integral part of the health care team. In addition to surveillance, the registered nurse assesses, refers, and consults with the NPs, physicians, and ancillary team members to obtain the intervention that best meets patient needs. This process allows the program to treat more patients cost-effectively and efficiently.

DISSEMINATION TO SYSTEM HOSPITALS

The transitional care model, with the integration of the interventions described earlier, was disseminated to 2 additional hospitals within the health care system: a large metropolitan tertiary care center and a suburban community hospital. Patients diagnosed with pneumonia were also added to the program population. In addition to decreasing 30-day hospital readmission, the goals expanded to include the barriers noted earlier: decreasing the cost of care, identifying appropriate patients, and assigning interventions based on predicted risk of readmission. The team expanded to include additional NP staff, a social worker, pharmacist, registered nurse, and administrative support.

Interdisciplinary Team

The addition of the dedicated social worker, pharmacist, registered nurse, and administrative support has been invaluable. The most notable achievement has been the expanded ability of the NP to oversee patients. In the original transitional care model, an NP could oversee a maximum of approximately 16 patients. In the new transitional care model, an NP can oversee approximately 60 patients with the support of the team.

Changes in Workflow

The new model has required significant changes in workflow for the NP staff.

With the implementation of appropriate patient identification, referrals are now generated by inpatient social workers and care coordinators, who remain integral partners. All new patient notifications occur within the patient identification and predictive risk tool, which generate an electronic message notifying the transitional care team of potential program candidates. Documentation regarding the status of a referral is captured within the tool and is accessible to all team members for review and care coordination. Internal validation of the tool reveals 95% to 99% specificity.

Risk Stratification and Remote Monitoring

Internal data suggest that predictive risk accuracy and acceptance of remote monitoring is high. The team escalates the level of intervention for less than 5% of patients, and remote monitoring allows other team members to intervene, often successfully, before escalating to the NP or the primary care provider. The remote monitoring includes indicators for frailty, depression, and patient satisfaction, which the team is working to maximally integrate into current practice.

Weekly Team Meetings

The transitional team meets weekly. Meetings begin with a review of the previous week's data, led by the medical director; then each NP present an update on their assigned high-risk patients currently followed by the team, and then lower-risk patients for whom concern exists are discussed. The electronic medical record is reviewed and rounding notes are written. Remote monitoring data are reviewed simultaneously. Input from all involved team members and disciplines is sought to ensure evidence-based practices are in place. Ideas for change and practice improvement are encouraged. Although leadership is present, all team members are encouraged to have a strong and equal voice.

IMPLICATIONS FOR NURSING PRACTICE

Transitional care provides a platform for nurses to provide outstanding patient care, develop protocols based on evidence, assist in population management, lead intraprofessional teams, add to the body of nursing knowledge via transitional care research, and assume leadership roles in the hospitals and health care systems in which they work. For example, the NPs at the authors' institution are expected to be the transitional care model leaders for the hospitals they serve. Their role is not only patient care but also to understand the unique setting of care and the social and political mores within their hospitals. The NPs take lead on education related to changes in the transitional care model and are truly respected as clinical nursing leaders.

The transitional care team identified areas that require enhancement through knowledge, better collaboration, and coordination of care to improve outcomes. **Box 2** presents gaps in knowledge.

Box 2
Gaps in knowledge

Protocol-driven palliative care

Patient activation and engagement as it relates to recidivism and transitional care

Interventions for malnutrition, frailty, and depression during the transitional care period

Broad-based community support systems and engagement

Use of team members at their highest level of education and preparation

System integration between post-acute care providers, such as home health, hospice, and durable medical equipment providers

---

LESSONS LEARNED

The team did not anticipate expansion to be as challenging as it was. It became clear that outstanding teams must be nurtured, and that team building exercises and development are integral to success.

The time required for cultural change in different entities within the same large health care system was more than initially expected. The team particularly struggled with the patient identification and risk stratification tool, which requires the active engagement of all members of the team. If any team member shows a lack of engagement, the process has failed. The team has built in electronic feedback mechanisms to notify managers of areas of lesser engagement, which has helped manage the process. Hospitals and health care systems are advised to add more time than they anticipate when making significant changes in operational and clinical culture.

Legal barriers make full integration within and transparency across the health care system challenging. Sharing of vital health care information across all team members has not always been possible because of regulatory requirements and lack of job descriptions for positions between entities within the same health care system. Strong administrative leadership has been necessary to remove barriers to aide in delivery of care.

The nature of the work by the transitional care team has required a high degree of flexibility and efficiency. The team is continually required to make rapid changes to workflow, protocols, and other aspects of patient care. This challenge should be taken into account by hospitals considering these programs. The team has been well served by the ability to self-reflect on processes that work and those that do not, and the members understand their unique roles in the success or failure. An example of this is the original intent that the social worker and pharmacist be exclusively office-based. The NPs believed that these team members needed to be brought to the home in some circumstances to best meet patient needs. Subsequently, both social worker and pharmacist have made home visits, although this is not the norm.

The current fee-for-service structure does not well accommodate for changes in health care delivery methods. Providers generally are paid for their services and not for the quality of the services. Negotiating between the current payment structure and the structure probable in the future of health care is formidable.

SUMMARY

Health care in its current state continues to lack effectiveness and cost-effectiveness for the populations served. Health care providers and systems are challenged to develop models of care that deliver better care to more patients with chronic health care problems. Transitional care programs help avert the risk of rehospitalizations. However, current fee for service hinders sustainability of resource intensive services necessary in transitional care.

REFERENCES

1. Chronic Disease Prevention and Health Promotion. Centers for Disease Control and Prevention Web site. Available at: www.cdc.gov/chronicdisease/overview.htm. Accessed November 27, 2013.
2. Hall MJ, Levant S, DeFrances CJ. Hospitalization for congestive heart failure: United States, 2000–2010. NCHS data brief, no 108. Hyattsville (MD): National Center for Health Statistics; 2012.
3. Readmissions Reduction Program. Centers for Medicare & Medicaid Web site. Available at: http://www.cms.gov/medicare/medicare-fee-for-service-payment/

acuteinpatientPPS/readmissions-reduction-program.html. Accessed October 20, 2013.

4. Naylor MD, Brooten DA, Campbell RL, et al. Transitional care of older adults hospitalized with heart failure: a randomized controlled trial. J Am Geriatr Soc 2004; 52(5):675–84.

5. Coleman EA, Parry C, Chalmers S, et al. The care transitions intervention: results of a randomized controlled trial. Arch Intern Med 2006;166(17):1822–8.

6. Stauffer BD, Fullerton C, Fleming N, et al. Effectiveness and cost of a transitional care program for heart failure: a prospective study with concurrent controls. Arch Intern Med 2011;171(14):1238–43.

7. Amarasingham R, Moore BJ, Tabak YP, et al. An automated model to identify heart failure patients at risk for 30-day readmission or death using electronic medical record data. Med Care 2010;48(11):981–8.

8. Centers for Medicare and Medicaid Services recognize Mount Sinai for personalized follow-up care for Medicare patients. Available at: http://www. mountsinai.org/about-us/newsroom/press-releases/centers-for-medicare-and-medicaid-services-recognize-mount-sinai-for-personalized-follow-up-care-for-medicare-patients. Accessed October 20, 2013.

9. Pulse360. Transforming data in real-time for patient quality improvement. 360Fresh Web site. Available at: http://www.360fresh.com/offerings.html. Accessed October 20, 2013.

10. Inglis SC, Clark RA, McAlister FA, et al. Which components of heart failure programmes are effective: a systematic review and meta-analysis of the outcomes of structured telephone support or telemonitoring as the primary component of chronic heart failure management in 8323 patients: abridged Cochrane Review. Eur J Heart Fail 2011;13:1028–40.

11. Steventon A, Tunkel S, Blunt I, et al. Effect of telephone health coaching (Birmingham OwnHealth) on hospital use and associated costs: cohort study with matched controls. BMJ 2013;347:f4585. Available at: http://www.bmj.com/content/347/bmj.f4585?tab=metrics. Accessed October 20, 2013.

12. Our approach. Pharos Innovations Web site. Available at: http://www. pharosinnovations.com/our-approach.php. Accessed December 8, 2013.

13. Altfeld SJ, Shier GE, Rooney M, et al. Effects of an enhanced discharge planning intervention for hospitalized older adults: a randomized trial. Gerontologist 2013; 53(3):430–40.

14. Peek CJ, Baird MA, Coleman E. Primary care for patient complexity, not only disease. Fam Syst Health 2009;27(4):287–302.

15. Jencks SF, Williams MV, Coleman EA. Rehospitalizations among patients in the Medicare fee-for-service program. N Engl J Med 2009;360:1418–28.

16. Perry AJ, Golden RL, Rooney M, et al. Enhanced discharge planning program at Rush University Medical Center. In: Schraeder C, Shelton P, editors. Comprehensive care coordination for chronically ill adults. West Sussex (United Kingdom): John Wiley & Sons; 2011. p. 277–90.

17. Taylor Haynes K, Oberne A, Cawthon C, et al. Pharmacists' recommendations to improve care transitions. Ann Pharmacother 2012;46(9):1152–9.

The Application of the Acute Care Nurse Practitioner Role in a Cardiovascular Patient Population

CrossMark

Marygrace Hernandez-Leveille, PhD, RN, ACNP-BC[a],*,
Jasmiry D. Bennett, MS, RN, ACNP-BC[b],
Nicole Nelson, MSN, RN, ACNP-BC, CCRN[c]

KEYWORDS

• Acute care nurse practitioner • Acute care settings • Cardiovascular

KEY POINTS

- Acute care nurse practitioners (ACNP), in an acute care setting, have a vital role in the contribution to decreased length of hospital stay, readmission rates, and reduced patient mortality.
- The consensus model for APRN regulation allows for increased advanced practice registered nurse (APRN) care for patients.
- ACNPs serve as a liaison and advocate for patients and family members.
- The ACNP role combines evidence-based clinical practice with research, education, consultation, and leadership to provide high-quality, cost-effective patient care.

STATEMENT OF THE PROBLEM/IMPORTANCE OF THE PROBLEM

Currently, health care providers and health care systems are caught up in the whirlwind of the ever-changing state of the health care delivery systems. Much of this is owing to overarching political and hidden personal agendas. Health care systems are struggling to keep up with the evolving proposed health care changes while attempting to provide high-quality care, patient-centered holistic care, and equitable care in a cost-containment environment. Health care reform has empowered patients to have a voice in the delivery of their care. Providing true holistic patient-centered care is essential; patients' comments are publicized in consumer reports and are

Disclosure: The authors have nothing to disclose.
[a] Baylor University Medical Center at Dallas, 3500 Gaston Avenue, Dallas, TX 75246, USA;
[b] Baylor Heart and Vascular Hospital, 621 N Hall Street, Dallas, TX 75246, USA; [c] Dallas Pulmonary & Critical Care PA, 221 W. Colorado Boulevard Pav II Suite 525B, Dallas, TX 75208, USA
* Corresponding author.
E-mail address: Marygrace.leveille@baylorhealth.edu

Crit Care Nurs Clin N Am 26 (2014) 599–606
http://dx.doi.org/10.1016/j.ccell.2014.08.007
0899-5885/14/$ – see front matter © 2014 Elsevier Inc. All rights reserved.

the key to reimbursement for services rendered. Additionally, patients' and family members' access to social media provide the ability to instantaneously publicize any type of information, positive or negative, about a particular physician, nurse, or hospital. As we progress toward health care reform and address the challenges and barriers to quality and costs of care, the implementation of the Affordable Care Act, Accountable Care Organizations will be evaluating and admitting more insured patients and thus are responsible for providing safer, quality, patient-centered care to more patients than ever. Our society will no longer tolerate payment for quantity of services. Conversely, consumers will reward health care providers and health care systems for the value of the care provided and the quality of the care. The law supports patients in taking ownership of their health care. Patients and their family members need to be educated and equipped with the tools to be more engaged in the implementation of the interventions identified in the individual tailored plan of care for each patient.

The nursing profession is now being transformed to assist in the restructuring of health care systems that can offer safe, patient-centered, quality, accessible and affordable care as outlined by the Institute of Medicine report, "The Future of Nursing: Leading Change and Advancing Health."[1] Advanced practice registered nurses (APRNs) are being called to expand their roles and assist in closing the gap between insurance coverage and access to care. APRNs can fulfill their potential as providers as outlined by their educational preparation, training, national certification, and their states' specific scopes of practice.

More than ever, health care delivery systems need a multidisciplinary team approach to care for patients. The inclusion of acute care nurse practitioners (ACNPs) in this multidisciplinary approach to holistic, patient-centered care can bolster successful outcomes, such as decreased length of stay, decreased intensive care days, quality improvement initiatives, decreased readmission rates, fewer patient complications, and less patient morbidity and mortality in acute care settings. ACNPs are an invaluable investment for the hospital. ACNPs have the potential to assist hospitals in reducing costs while increasing quality outcomes.[2] The purpose of this review is to discuss the APRN evolving role in the climate of legislative health care change, emphasizing the expanding vital ACNP role in a cardiovascular setting, highlighted by a case study in which the ACNP was an integral part of the patient's successful outcome.

REVIEW OF THE LITERATURE

The role of the APRN evolved in the 1960s to fill a void to the nation-wide physician shortage. In the early 1990s, the utilization of APRNs was introduced into the hospital settings. APRNs can address a broad spectrum of patient issues from health promotion, diagnosing and prescribing for disease management, to coordination of care and, if required, palliative care. Each state within the United States has varying definitions and scopes of practice for an APRN. In addition to the national legislative health care changes, the nursing profession is addressing advanced practice registered nursing initiatives and regulatory processes for APRNs through the American Nurses Association. In July 2008, the document "Consensus Model for APRN Regulation: Licensure, Accreditation, Certification, and Education" was completed to address the standardization of regulatory processes for APRNs. This results in increased access to APRN care and increased mobility for APRNs. This association provides an APRN Regulatory Model that defines 4 advanced practice roles. These roles include nurse practitioner, nurse midwife, nurse anesthetist, and clinical nurse specialist.[3] Through these 4 roles, APRNs care for patients within 6 population foci. These include family/individual across lifespan, adult/gerontology, neonatal, pediatrics, women's health/gender-related, and psychiatric/mental health. From these populations, APRNs care for patients within a variety of specialties, including cardiology, orthopedics, oncology, and nephrology.[4]

The APRN consensus model includes 4 essential components of APRN regulation. In 2015, the American Nurses Association recommends full implementation of this APRN regulatory model and all recommendations. The acronym used to remember these important steps is *LACE*. The first letter, *L*, is for licensure. Once all educational requirements are completed and the APRN has successfully passed the national certification examination, the individual State Boards of Nursing grant the APRN authorization to practice within that state. The *A* is for accreditation, which is the official review and authorization by certification programs in nursing or nursing related programs or a recognized agency of educational degree. The Boards of Nursing defines APRNs as registered nurses who have completed an advanced educational program that is accredited by a national organization and that prepares them for 1 of the 4 advanced practice roles. During this role transformation, the registered nurse is expected to acquire advanced skills and clinical knowledge to provide more autonomous direct and indirect patient care after graduation. The *C* is for certification, which is the official recognition of the skills, knowledge, and experience based on the achievement of professional standards. An APRN demonstrates clinical competence by passing a national certification examination that measures population-focused competencies, the advanced practice role, and demonstrating continued competence by maintaining certification or performing recertification. The American Nurses Association supports professional certification, because the individual state licensing boards do not regulate APRNs at their specialty level. The *E* is for education. This is the official preparation that APRNs receive in either graduate degree programs or postgraduate certificate programs. These programs must be accredited by a nursing or nursing-related organization that is recognized by either the Council for Higher Education Accreditation or the US Department of Education.[5] Currently, individual state Boards of Nursing determine the criteria that are sufficient to achieve an APRN status, such as the number of clinical hours during the nursing program; the number of didactic hours specific to pathophysiology, pharmacotherapeutics, and advanced health assessment; the number of clinical practicum hours; and theoretic and clinical role preparation.

The individual State Boards of Nursing identify an APRN's scope of practice as having advanced practice education within a designated specialty and role, identifying legal implications and maintaining compliance with the individual Board of Nursing and Nurse Practice Act, and following scope of practice statements issued by advanced practice nursing organizations and national professional specialty organizations. The board further specifies professional and individual scopes of practice. The nurse practitioner's professional scope of practice is the first component in defining their scope of practice, because advanced practice nursing organizations and national specialty organizations provide a broad scope of practice for each type of role within each specialty. This depends on the nurse practitioner's function, role, practice setting, and the population they care for. In the individual scope of practice, the nurse practitioner's formal education becomes their foundation. Their scope of practice becomes limitless as they grow their clinical experience in various practice settings, through continuing education, formal course work completion, and the evolution of health care. The APRN is liable to know and practice within their professional and individual scopes of practice.[6] The current challenges for APRNs pertain to several constraints of prescriptive authority within the various states, the numerous versions of scopes of practice from state to state, the issue of autonomous practice and collaborating practice, reimbursement, and education preparation standardization.

The ACNP role evolved from an adult nurse practitioner role to include hospital-based practice to care for inpatient acutely ill patients. Since the first ACNP certification examination, which was established in 1995, ACNPs have been a vital component of providing care to a variety of acutely ill patients in a variety of settings such as intensive care units, tertiary care settings, trauma centers, and specialty medicine areas such as oncology, gastroenterology, and interventional radiology.[7] ACNPs are empowered, accountable, and competent to make high-level decisions, making appropriate assessments to contribute to the care of an acutely ill patient.

ACNPs are prepared to assess and stabilize critically ill patients through critical thinking skills acquired during the required clinical hours during the course of their advanced educational preparation. The developing ACNP role offers an opportunity to expand functions within the scopes of practice as allowed by the respective state boards of nursing. Although many ACNPs report high levels to extremely high levels of autonomy, levels of autonomy and prescriptive authority can vary from state to state and the individual practice setting.[8] The ACNP role requires the integration of knowledge, clinical experience, and critical thinking skills, as well as the ability to comprehensively assess the patient to adequately determine the differential diagnoses.[9] ACNPs are employed in a variety of settings performing clinical skills, such as central and peripheral line insertion, intubation, ventilator management, interpretation of laboratory and radiography, mechanical circulatory support devices, and first assisting in surgical procedures.[10] Laschinger and colleagues[11] assert that ACNPs in acute care settings have greater job satisfaction because of the increased levels of autonomy. ACNPs in acute care settings reported increased satisfaction in their role because of their autonomy and collaborative care and were highly skillful and competent while managing patients requiring high-level, comprehensive care.[8,9]

First and foremost, ACNPs are patient advocates. The ultimate goal of the ACNP is to provide the best evidence-based care possible and ACNPs have been proven to be successful in numerous departments.[12] This goal can be achieved by the ACNP actively engaged with the patient and family members, and also working with an interdisciplinary team to formulate a patient-specific plan of care tailored to address the physical, emotional, and psychosocial needs of the patient.[13] Although one would argue that there is not a "typical" day for an ACNP, the ACNP is an integral part of co-ordination of care; enhancing communication between the nursing staff, physicians, other clinicians, and ancillary departments; educating nursing staff and patients; and facilitating processes required for discharge to either the patients' home, rehabilitation center, or skilled nursing unit.[12,14,15] On a daily basis, in an effort to reduce hospital length of stay, mortality and morbidity, and hospital readmission rates, the ACNP is constantly evaluating avenues to contain cost while providing safe and efficient care, increase patient satisfaction, and ensure the plan of care comprises action plans to ensure patient safety.[8,10,12,16,17] As a result of the ACNP's consistent vigilance over these clinical indicators, patients who received care from ACNPs had the same clinical outcomes as patients who were managed by hospitalist-led care.[14,17]

This case study highlights the role of an ACNP caring for an acutely ill patient hospitalized over 70 days. On a daily basis, the ACNP communicated and partnered with the nursing team, physicians, and ancillary staff to organize care to ensure the safety of the patient during the hospitalization. As in this case, the key to optimal care is communication, trust, staff confidence, and the mutual shared respect between the ACNP and the rest of the health care team. The consistent attentiveness of the ACNP and the interdisciplinary team was crucial.

CASE STUDY

A 35-year-old Hispanic man presented to the emergency room with complaints of chest pain and shortness of breath. He had a medical history of uncontrolled diabetes, hypertension, end-stage renal disease on hemodialysis, and a surgical history of right lower extremity transmetatarsal amputation, left below-the-knee amputation, left arteriovenous fistula creation with thrombectomy, and multiple fistula revisions. He was hypotensive, tachycardic, febrile, acidotic, and hypoxic. His initial workup consisted of a computed tomography angiogram to rule out a pulmonary embolus; it was negative. Laboratory evaluation revealed an elevated white blood cell count (>20) and a hemoglobin of 7, with a hematocrit of 21. The electrocardiogram demonstrated sinus tachycardia with no acute electrocardiographic changes. The echocardiogram revealed a large mitral valve vegetation with severe mitral regurgitation. His primary admitting diagnosis was acute endocarditis with severe mitral regurgitation. Owing to his declining state, he was fluid resuscitated and vasopressors were initiated; intubation was required for oxygenation support. His emergent presentation warranted an emergent mitral valve replacement with cardiothoracic surgery.

Despite his initial critical presentation, his postoperative course was uneventful. As a result of adequate oxygenation and a stable hemodynamic state, he was successfully extubated and weaned off the vasopressors. On postoperative day 4, the patient started complaining of left lower extremity pain. Upon assessment by the ACNP, his left lower extremity was mottled, and a femoral pulse or signal was appreciated. An arterial duplex revealed an arterial thrombus and he was emergently taken for thrombectomy. Once he was stabilized postoperatively, anticoagulation was initiated. However, the next day he complained of right hand pain and, upon additional evaluation, an arterial duplex revealed a thrombosed radial artery. As a result, he underwent right radial artery thrombectomy. As a result of his infective endocarditis, remnants continued to shower microembolisms. His condition continued to deteriorate as he then developed profound hypotension with systolic blood pressures of 60 to 70 mm Hg that did not respond to fluid resuscitation. It was at this point that the ACNP was approached by the nursing staff to evaluate this patient and work collaboratively with the cardiovascular surgeons, cardiologists, and nephrologist to manage the multisystem issues at hand.

In addition to microembolisms and emergent surgeries, the patient has still required daily hemodialysis for 4 consecutive days. However, with a differential diagnosis of hypovolemia, he continued to be profoundly hypovolemic requiring colloid fluid resuscitation. Despite adequate fluid resuscitation, the patient remained hypotensive and hemodialysis was placed on hold. After a team discussion between the ACNP, cardiovascular surgeon, and nephrologist, an echocardiogram was ordered to further assess ventricular function and structural components to further ascertain the basis for the profound hypotension. The echocardiogram revealed large amount of fluid around the pericardium consistent with cardiac tamponade and the patient subsequently suffered a cardiac arrest. He was taken emergently to the operating room and underwent pericardial window. After an uneventful postoperative recovery, he was transferred back to the cardiac step-down unit.

The patient started to deteriorate a few days after having been transferred to the step-down unit; he was becoming intermittently hypotensive. The ACNP examined the patient and noted the patient to have purulent drainage from his left lower extremity above-the-knee amputation. The ACNP consulted a vascular surgeon and a surgical resident was assigned to complete a bedside debridement. The left lower extremity above-the-knee amputation incision was opened at the bedside and copious purulent drainage was expressed from the wound followed by a packed wet-to-dry dressing. The next day, during the ACNP's daily physical assessment of the patient, the ACNP did not appreciate any improvement in the patient's level of pain or wound site, and again contacted the vascular surgeon for further evaluation. As a result of the vascular surgeon bedside assessment and concurring with the ACNP's assessment of the patients' left lower extremity wound, the patient was taken to the operating room later that day for further debridement and washout of the left lower extremity wound. The patient sustained poor circulation to his left lower extremity and, despite multiple attempts to restore the circulation to the extremity, he required a higher above-the-knee amputation necessitating multiple additional revisions and debridement of infected wound. Despite these efforts, the left above-the-knee amputation wound was not healing. The ACNP spent many hours explaining to the patient, family members, and the nursing staff the gravity of the situation and the need to consult the vascular surgeon again given the presentation of the wound and the signs and symptoms of sepsis reoccurring. The ACNP again contacted the vascular surgeon who in turn consulted an orthopedic surgeon for hip disarticulation. After the hip disarticulation was completed, the patient recovered well. Daily information was provided to the patient and the family members.

While the patient was recovering on the step-down unit, he started to experience episodes of shortness of breath requiring increased FiO_2 support to maintain adequate oxygenation. The ACNP discussed with the nursing staff his vital signs, oxygenation and nursing physical assessment. Subsequent to the ACNP's physical assessment findings, a chest x-ray was ordered and revealed a large right pleural effusion. The ACNP communicated these findings to cardiothoracic surgeon, who suggested a thoracentesis be completed by interventional radiology. In an attempt to remove some of the fluid, hemodialysis was ordered by the cardiovascular surgeon. Later that day, the patient experienced respiratory arrest and was intubated, therefore requiring a transfer back to the intensive care unit. A thoracentesis was performed with more than 1.5 L extracted. Once his pulmonary status stabilized and he was adequately able to oxygenate, he was extubated and transferred to the step-down unit where he continued to recover.

As the interdisciplinary team waited for the right hand to demarcate and show signs of necrosis, physical assessment and hemodynamic changes consistent with sepsis were once again present. Upon examination, the ACNP noted his midsternal incision dehisced distally with minor exposure of his midsternal wire surrounded by purulent drainage. In addition, the patient also complained of right wrist and thumb pain. Through the coordination of the ACNP, the cardiothoracic surgeon and the plastic surgeon combined their operations and the patient was then taken to the operating room, where he underwent removal of midsternal wire and amputation of his right thumb with debridement of his wrist. A wound Vac was placed on the forearm, right hand, and midsternal area. The patient currently continues to recuperate at day 70 in the hospital with plans of discharge in the near future to a rehabilitation center. The ACNP continues to coordinate care with the physicians, nurses, respiratory therapy, physical therapy, and occupational therapy specialists to ensure optimization of his care before discharge. Care coordination discharge nurses and social workers will also be involved to ensure the continuum of care and progress of the patient's outpatient recovery.

The ACNP has been the main constant in this patient's care throughout his hospitalization. The ACNP has formed a personal bond with the patient and his family. The patient is no longer "Mr So and So" in room 207. He is a part of the ACNP's daily life. The ACNP has invested her clinical, medical expertise with her personal nuances and a true caring human bond has been formed. Despite this patient's multiple comorbidities, circulatory issues requiring emergent surgical interventions, respiratory deteriorations, and sepsis, coordination of care, as spearheaded by the ACNP, with other clinicians and multiple disciplines has allowed this patient to live with a potential to go home and live a promising life.

Although health care delivery systems are faced with the financial concerns of increasing cost for providing care, it is unethical to withhold treatment owing to a patients' increased length of stay in the hospital. In this case, the primary concern of the ACNP and the physicians was to provide the best care possible. When appropriate, avenues to shave cost and minimize patient exposure to unnecessary procedures and medications were evaluated. This was evident in the ACNPs coordination of 2 surgeries to limit anesthesia exposure time when the patient required hand/thumb surgery and removal of the midsternal wire. In this case study and all other patient care opportunities, the nurse practitioner is the liaison and advocate for the patient and family members.

CHALLENGES AND BARRIERS

Although the ACNP role can be extremely rewarding in many ways, challenges and barriers exist. One of the goals of the consensus model is to offer uniformity in state APRN regulatory issues and prescriptive authority. The resolution of these primary issues will allow for increased access of care for patients utilizing APRN's in their full capacity. To achieve this increase in access of health care for all Americans, there must be an evolving legislative movement at both the federal and state levels. State-imposed limitations within the scope of practice hinder APRN resource utilization and contribute to increased health care costs. As a result of these incongruent practices, physicians and society are confused with the APRN role and inconsistent acceptance from other health care providers as well. In addition, the ACNP will be required to continually define their role, privileges, and defend their role for credentialing purposes. Depending on the state and practice site, an ACNP can potentially be underutilized or overutilized. An ACNP can potentially be in a high-intensity role and in a work environment where participation in research and quality initiatives is expected. However, time constraints from patient management limits the ACNP in full engagement in these other important initiatives. Additionally, billing and reimbursement issues, at times, continue to surface as controversial issues to a practicing ACNP either in private practice or an acute care setting. As the ACNP role evolves and legislative initiatives continue to surface, resolution of these issues are on the horizon.

SUMMARY

The ACNP has been defined as being knowledgeable in assessment, differential diagnosis, clinical reasoning, ordering diagnostics tests and treatments, executing patient-centered management plans, and prescribing medications. This role is vital in an acute care environment because the nurse practitioner unites expert, evidence-based clinical practice with research, education, consultation, and leadership. The case study reviewed in this paper demonstrated the ACNP role of providing prompt attention to early deterioration warning signs resulting in improved coordination patient care and increased patient satisfaction. The inclusion of ACNPs in a cardiovascular patient setting has proven to be effective with regard to decreasing hospital length of stay, reduction of cost to the patient and the hospital, and increasing nursing and patient satisfaction.

REFERENCES

1. National Research Council. The future of nursing: leading change, advancing health. Washington, DC: The National Academies Press; 2010. Available at: http://www.nap.edu/catalog/12956.html. Accessed December 11, 2013.
2. Liego M, Loomis J, Van Leuven K, et al. Improving outcomes through the proper implementation of acute care nurse practitioners. J Nurs Adm 2014;44(1):47–50. http://dx.doi.org/10.1097/NNA.0000000000000020.
3. APRN Consensus Work Group & the National Council of State Boards of Nursing APRN Advisory Committee. Consensus model for APRN regulation: licensure, accreditation, certification, and education. Silver Spring (MD): American Nurses Association; 2008. Available at: http://www.nursingworld.org/cmissuebrief. Accessed December 11, 2013.
4. Woolbert L, Ziegler B, Taylor L. A guide for APRN practice in Texas. Cedar Park (TX): Coalition for Nurses in Advanced Practice; 2013. Available at: http://www.cnaptexas.org/?page=APRNGuide4thEdition. Accessed March 19, 2014.
5. Summers L. Consensus model for APRN regulation: licensure, accreditation, certification, education presentation for constituent member associations of the American Nurses Association. Silver Spring (MD): American Nurses Association; 2009. Available at: http://www.nursingworld.org/cmpowerpoint. Accessed October 5, 2013.
6. Texas Board of Nursing. Guidelines for determining APN scope of practice. Austin (TX): Texas Board of Nursing; 2005. Available at: http://www.bon.texas.gov/practice/apn-scopeofpractice.html. Accessed October 5, 2013.
7. Kleinpell R. Reports of role descriptions of acute care nurse practitioners. AACN Clin Issues 1998;9(2):290–5.
8. Cajulis CB, Fitzpatrick JJ. Levels of autonomy of nurse practitioners in an acute care setting. J Am Acad Nurse Pract 2007;19(10):500–7.
9. Kleinpell R. Evolving role descriptions of the acute care nurse practitioner. Crit Care Nurs Q 1999;21(4):9–15.
10. Rosenthal L, Guerrasio G. Acute care nurse practitioner as hospitalist: role description. Crit Care Nurse 2010;20(2):21–5. Available at: http://www.aacn.org/WD/CETests/Media/CG02103.pdf. Accessed October 5, 2013.
11. Laschinger HK, Almost J, Tuer-Hodes D. Workplace empowerment and magnet hospital characteristics. J Nurs Adm 2003;33:410–22. Available at: http://www.nursingcenter.com/lnc/journalarticle?Article_ID=420271. Accessed December 11, 2013.
12. Moore H. The impact of the cardiac surgical nurse practitioner role on the ward. Br J Card Nurs 2012;7(12):604–5.
13. Sidani S, Doran D, Porter H, et al. Outcomes of nurse practitioners in acute care: an exploration. Internet J Adv Nurs Pract 2006;8(1). Available at: http://ispub.com/IJANP/8/1/12232. Accessed June 23, 2013.
14. Tedesco J. Acute care nurse practitioners in transplantation: adding value to your program. Prog Transplant 2011;21(4):278–83.
15. Casida JM, Pastor J. Practice pattern and professional issues of nurse practitioners in mechanical circulatory support programs in the United States: a survey report. Prog Transplant 2012;22(3):229–36. http://dx.doi.org/10.7182/pit2012503.
16. Fry M. Literature review of the impact of nurse practitioners in critical care services. Nurs Crit Care 2011;16(2):58–66.
17. Goldie CL, Prodan-Bhalla N, Mackay M. Nurse practitioners in postoperative cardiac surgery: are they effective? Can J Cardiovasc Nurs 2012;22(4):8–15.

Index

NOTE: Page numbers of article titles are in **boldface** type.

United States Postal Service

Statement of Ownership, Management, and Circulation
(All Periodicals Publications Except Requestor Publications)

1. Publication Title	2. Publication Number	3. Filing Date
Critical Care Nursing Clinics of North America	0 0 6 - 2 7 3	9/14/14

4. Issue Frequency	5. Number of Issues Published Annually	6. Annual Subscription Price
Mar, Jun, Sep, Dec	4	$150.00

7. Complete Mailing Address of Known Office of Publication (Not printer) (Street, city, county, state, and ZIP+4®)

Elsevier Inc.
360 Park Avenue South
New York, NY 10010-1710

Contact Person
Stephen R. Bushing

Telephone (Include area code)
215-239-3688

8. Complete Mailing Address of Headquarters or General Business Office of Publisher (Not printer)

Elsevier Inc., 360 Park Avenue South, New York, NY 10010-1710

9. Full Names and Complete Mailing Addresses of Publisher, Editor, and Managing Editor (Do not leave blank)

Publisher (Name and complete mailing address)

Linda Belfus, Elsevier Inc., 1600 John F. Kennedy Blvd., Suite 1800, Philadelphia, PA 19103-2899

Editor (Name and complete mailing address)

Kerry Holland, Elsevier Inc., 1600 John F. Kennedy Blvd., Suite 1800, Philadelphia, PA 19103-2899

Managing Editor (Name and complete mailing address)

Adrianne Brigido, Elsevier Inc., 1600 John F. Kennedy Blvd., Suite 1800, Philadelphia, PA 19103-2899

10. Owner (Do not leave blank. If the publication is owned by a corporation, give the name and address of the corporation immediately followed by the names and addresses of all stockholders owning or holding 1 percent or more of the total amount of stock. If not owned by a corporation, give the names and addresses of the individual owners. If owned by a partnership or other unincorporated firm, give its name and address as well as those of each individual owner. If the publication is published by a nonprofit organization, give its name and address.)

Full Name	Complete Mailing Address
Wholly owned subsidiary of	1600 John F. Kennedy Blvd., Ste. 1800
Reed/Elsevier, US holdings	Philadelphia, PA 19103-2899

11. Known Bondholders, Mortgagees, and Other Security Holders Owning or Holding 1 Percent or More of Total Amount of Bonds, Mortgages, or Other Securities. If none, check box. ☐ None

Full Name	Complete Mailing Address
N/A	

12. Tax Status (For completion by nonprofit organizations authorized to mail at nonprofit rates) (Check one)
The purpose, function, and nonprofit status of this organization and the exempt status for federal income tax purposes:
☐ Has Not Changed During Preceding 12 Months
☐ Has Changed During Preceding 12 Months (Publisher must submit explanation of change with this statement)

PS Form 3526, August 2012 (Page 1 of 3 (Instructions Page 3)) PSN 7530-01-000-9931 PRIVACY NOTICE: See our Privacy policy in www.usps.com

---

13. Publication Title	14. Issue Date for Circulation Data Below
Critical Care Nursing Clinics of North America	June 2014

15. Extent and Nature of Circulation		Average No. Copies Each Issue During Preceding 12 Months	No. Copies of Single Issue Published Nearest to Filing Date
a. Total Number of Copies (Net press run)		484	441
b. Paid Circulation (By Mail and Outside the Mail)	(1) Mailed Outside-County Paid Subscriptions Stated on PS Form 3541. (Include paid distribution above nominal rate, advertiser's proof copies, and exchange copies)	331	290
	(2) Mailed In-County Paid Subscriptions Stated on PS Form 3541 (Include paid distribution above nominal rate, advertiser's proof copies, and exchange copies)		
	(3) Paid Distribution Outside the Mails Including Sales Through Dealers and Carriers, Street Vendors, Counter Sales, and Other Paid Distribution Outside USPS®	59	54
	(4) Paid Distribution by Other Classes Mailed Through the USPS (e.g. First-Class Mail®)		
c. Total Paid Distribution (Sum of 15b (1), (2), (3), and (4))	▶	390	334
d. Free or Nominal Rate Distribution (By Mail and Outside the Mail)	(1) Free or Nominal Rate Outside-County Copies Included on PS Form 3541	36	38
	(2) Free or Nominal Rate In-County Copies Included on PS Form 3541		
	(3) Free or Nominal Rate Copies Mailed at Other Classes Through the USPS (e.g. First-Class Mail)		
	(4) Free or Nominal Rate Distribution Outside the Mail (Carriers or other means)		
e. Total Free or Nominal Rate Distribution (Sum of 15d (1), (2), (3) and (4))	▶	36	38
f. Total Distribution (Sum of 15c and 15e)	▶	426	382
g. Copies not Distributed (See instructions to publishers #4 (page #3))	▶	58	59
h. Total (Sum of 15f and g)	▶	484	441
i. Percent Paid (15c divided by 15f times 100)	▶	91.55%	90.05%

16. Total circulation includes electronic copies. Report circulation on PS Form 3526-X worksheet.

17. Publication of Statement of Ownership
If the publication is a general publication, publication of this statement is required. Will be printed in the December 2014 issue of this publication.

18. Signature and Title of Editor, Publisher, Business Manager, or Owner

[signature]

Stephen R. Bushing – Inventory Distribution Coordinator

Date
September 14, 2014

I certify that all information furnished on this form is true and complete. I understand that anyone who furnishes false or misleading information on this form or who omits material or information requested on the form may be subject to criminal sanctions (including fines and imprisonment) and/or civil sanctions (including civil penalties).

PS Form 3526, August 2012 (Page 2 of 3)

Printed and bound by CPI Group (UK) Ltd, Croydon, CR0 4YY

03/10/2024

01040487-0020